Fitting Fitness In

to Stay Fit, Sharp & Independent as You Age

"One thing I particularly appreciate about all of Holly's exercise programs is that she demonstrates genuine concern for the senior citizens in her classes. She listens when we ask questions or ask for help with particular muscles or areas of our bodies. She attends classes and seminars to stay up to date. To keep things interesting Holly has fun sayings like, "Tighten your core and you can do more" or "Motion is lotion". These are repeated often in exercise class and I find myself repeating them to myself even away from class to remind myself of the benefits of Holly's teaching. Holly Kouvo has made a noticeable difference in my life.

Thank you for being such a valuable resource to your active agers!

~Chris F

THE FITTING FITNESS IN® SERIES

Fitting Fitness In to Stay Fit, Sharp & Independent as You Age

Holly Kouvo

CERTIFIED BRAIN HEALTH TRAINER,
FUNCTIONAL AGING SPECIALIST & NUTRITION SPECIALIST

ISBN: 978-097893563-4 (Softcover)
ISBN: 978-097893564-1 (Kindle)

Cover & Interior Design & Typesetting:
Desktop Miracles, Inc.

Holly Kouvo
http://www.fittingfitnessin.com/fitting-fitness-in-book/
www.HollyKouvo.com

Limits of Liability and Disclaimer of Warranty

The author and publisher shall not be liable for your misuse of this material. This book is strictly for informational and educational purposes.

Warning—Disclaimer

The purpose of this book is to educate and entertain. The author and/or publisher do not guarantee that anyone following these techniques, suggestions, tips, ideas, or strategies will become successful. The author and/or publisher shall have neither liability nor responsibility to anyone with respect to any loss or damage caused, or alleged to be caused, directly or indirectly by the information contained in this book.

To my clients,
Fitness is the fountain of youth.
Keep Moving!

Acknowledgments

I want to acknowledge the support and encouragement my husband has given me while I wrote this book. I would also like to thank my friend Robin who let me hide away at her cottage to work on my book without interruptions. Thank you to Dianne who kept me accountable throughout this process. Thank you to my first readers for your thoughts and feedback.

Thank you.

Contents

Foreword

DAN RITCHIE

Co-founder Functional Aging Institute

I am really excited that you have decided to pick up Holly's book. As I have worked with thousands of active-agers I have become convinced many of us are going to live 10, even 15 years longer than we ever would have guessed! In fact, you may have some family members now that you have all been surprised have made it into their 90s or beyond. While living to 90 or even 100 may sound like a nice thing, and it can be, it can also be very challenging if you do not do it well. I want you for a moment to consider what you want your life to be like at age 85? Do you want to be fit, strong, healthy, vibrant, socially engaged, and have a sharp mind? Or do you want to be frail, weak, dependent on others, no longer able to drive, struggling with your balance and cognitive abilities? You see we really all are training for that 85th birthday the question in front of you now as you begin this book.....are you training to be fit or frail at 85? Of course, no one really aspires to be frail or dependent, but often we don't take our training for age 85 seriously in our 50s, 60s, or 70s. While we hear it said it is never too late to get started on an exercise program and healthier lifestyle it sure is helpful to get started sooner, before you have osteoporosis, or cognitive issues. As we age, we can lose so much muscle, so much power, so much bone density that it is hard to build that all back if you put it off until you have more time. And when exactly are you going to find more time? The fact that you have picked up Holly's book already puts you in the top 5% of active agers. Learning from a Functional Aging Specialist the strategies you need to improve your balance, your brain health and your overall health and fitness will put you way ahead of the game. And let's be honest we are all in this game of life, and while it is going to end for all of us, we want to finish the race strong.

I want to share two quick stories with you. In case you have picked up this book and are worried it might already be too late for you, did you wait too long, can your aging trajectory be changed, yes it can. Don came to me at the age of 88 years old, and he described himself as a tottering old man. Now 88 probably is reasonable to call someone an old man, he had already outlived most of his peers, but Don wanted more in life. Don realized as an older grandfather he was going to miss out on high school graduations and college graduations and maybe someday weddings as he could barely handle traveling anymore. When he first came to meet with me, he walked like an old man, he had the posture of an old man, he moved slowly and was almost shuffling, he certainly looked like a fall risk waiting to happen. And Don, like so many his age was starting to wonder can anything even be done to help me? Well six months later and Don is slamming medicine balls, and slinging battle ropes and bear-crawling around the gym....you would have thought for a minute it was his 70 year old younger brother! At the age of 90 Don wrote me a letter I'll never forget (hopefully similar to one you will write Holly someday). In that letter Don shared we had forever changed his life and his 90s would never be the same! He had already traveled and seen a grandchild graduate high school and fully believed he would be able to see them all graduate and that his 90s could be healthy and vibrant!

Lastly, I want to encourage you after reading this book to think about what could be, what could come, what might you still be called to do in this world? My grandmother I will never forget felt called to teach English as a second language in Pakistan to Afghan refugee women. She had a strong affinity for these women as my grandfather built a hospital in Afghanistan in the 1970s. So, at the young age of 80 she headed off to Pakistan for 3 years. I don't remember anyone ever questioning whether she could do it physically, emotionally or cognitively. I think a few wondered why don't you just take it easy and be a grandma you know like in a rocking chair? I said of course you should go, you have people to help and serve, you can't stay here like a caged bird you are meant to fly. The fact that she was 80 was simply not part of the decision. Are you ready for what life might bring you at age 75, 80 or beyond? Dream bigger and be ready. Holly has all the tools for you to live your best decades still to come, now the rest as they say is up to you.

Introduction

What would you do if one day you couldn't get up off the toilet alone?

Is getting dressed, climbing stairs, or standing up from a chair starting to feel harder than it should?

Did you watch your parents go from vibrant to dependent – and wonder if you're next?

Are you slowly slipping into the same decline you swore you'd never repeat?

What if today is the strongest you'll ever be – unless you choose to change something?

I want to help you avoid being dependent on others and stay active and functional longer in your life.

While we can't control everything about our health, there are a lot of things you can do to live a healthier longer life.

I want you to have a long healthspan.

What is the meaning of **healthspan** versus **lifespan**? Lifespan is the total number of years we live whereas, healthspan is how many of those years we remain healthy and free from disease.

This book is accessible and filled with simple lifestyle changes that you can implement now to keep you thriving as you age.

This book is divided into three pillars of focus: Exercise, Nutrition, and Brain & Balance.

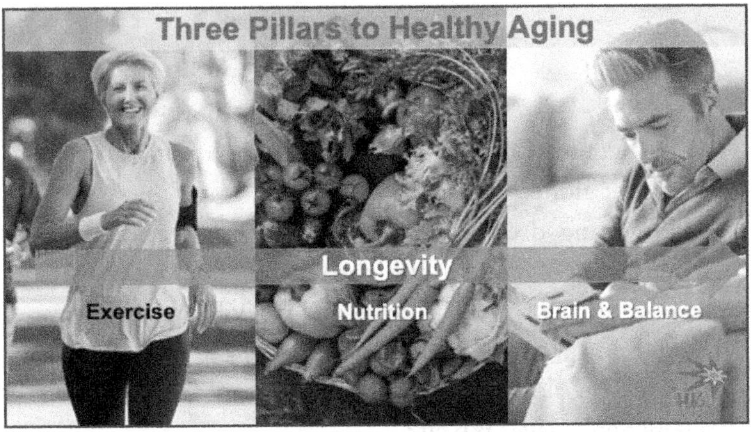

These are the 3 pillars you should invest in to improve your longevity. These will help you live more actively now and later in life.

Investing in these pillars now and continuing to invest in them will keep you fit, sharp, living independently, and more energized.

About Holly

I am a Functional Aging Specialist, Brain Health Trainer, Nutrition Specialist, Author, Speaker, and founder of Fitting Fitness In®. I have been working in the Fitness Industry over 20 years. I started my fitness business after working in high tech for 13 years.

I have been teaching my Brains & Balance class for over 10 years. Balance is so important as falls are a leading cause of hospitalizations in the US. One fall can change your life. We need to work on our balance every day. Later in this book I will give you easy practical exercises you can do at home to improve your balance. Don't wait until you are 80 years old to work on your balance. I have worked on balance with clients as young as 25 years old.

Keeping your brain active and healthy is very important as you age. With computers and calculators doing so much for us now, we haven't been using our brains as much. It's important to give your brain a workout, as well as your body. I have enjoyed seeing the difference in my class participants after working on balance and brain activities. They become much sharper and quicker in their responses.

Why I am writing this book?

My mom was diagnosed with Alzheimer's disease at 69 years old. It was a very hard time and my father had a hard time accepting the diagnosis. Since Alzheimer's is hereditary, that put me at a 50% chance of getting Alzheimer's. When I asked my mom's doctor "What can I do to help prevent getting this disease?", he said exercise, eat healthy foods, don't smoke, and don't drink alcohol. He emphasized **Stay active!**

Once all my siblings and I moved out of the house, my mom was not very active. She sat on the couch and read books. She passed away at the age of 87. That was 18 years of watching her cognitively decline.

My father had heart disease, he had a few heart attacks, a triple bypass, and a heart valve replacement. All of my siblings have heart disease. **I DO NOT.** My brother died of a heart attack at 67 years old.

When people ask me why I do what I do, I say I am living proof that you can take control of your health at any age. According to a study published online in the journal BMJ Evidence Based Medicine, a healthy lifestyle can offset the effects of life-shortening genes, your DNA, by over 60%.

I am writing this book because I believe that and I live that lifestyle! I should have heart disease. I do not. I want to motivate you to make some lifestyle changes that will help you to age with good health and energy.

Some words and terms I use in this book may be unfamiliar to you. They will be defined in the chapter they are used, but can also be found in the Glossary at the end of the book.

What will you get from reading this book?

After reading this book you will:

- Understand what lifestyle habits will help you live longer.
- Learn how you can avoid some diseases
- Know simple exercises to improve your balance.
- Master strategies to help you thrive later in life.
- Be motivated to start incorporating some of the simple lifestyle changes you have learned.

1

Become an Active Ager!

"Holly is an inspiration to
all of her "Active Agers".
Her dedication, drive and lively spirit
keeps us going!"

~ FRED F

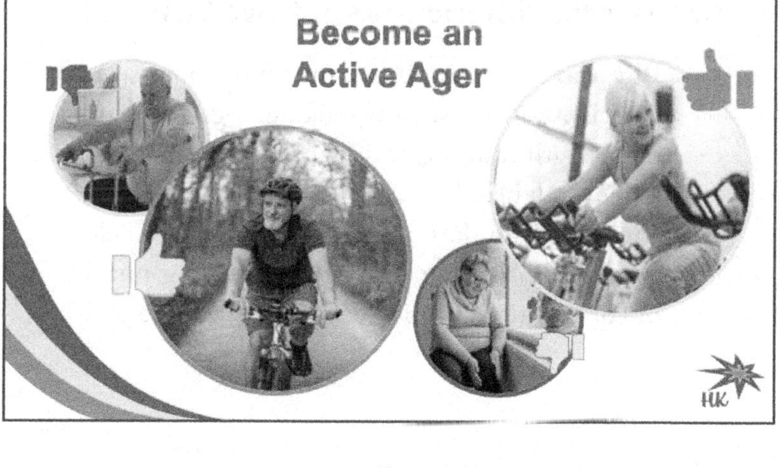

An active ager is someone (in the later stages of life) who prioritizes physical, mental, emotional, and social well-being to lead a fulfilling and engaged lifestyle. Instead of slowing down or becoming sedentary as they age, active agers embrace opportunities for growth, health, and contribution, adapting positively to the changes that come with aging.

Active aging focuses on quality of life as individuals grow older. It shifts the narrative from aging being about decline to viewing it as a period for continued growth, contribution, and joy.

This concept of active agers aligns with global efforts, such as the World Health Organization's (WHO) Active Aging Framework, which emphasizes independence, participation, and dignity for older adults. The WHO's active ageing framework is a call to action for policymakers, organizations, and individuals to create a world where older adults can thrive and contribute to society throughout their lives.

These are the characteristics of Active Agers:

- **Physical Activity:** They maintain or adopt regular exercise routines, such as walking, yoga, swimming, or strength training, to support mobility, strength, and overall health.
- **Mental Stimulation:** They engage in lifelong learning, hobbies, or activities like reading, puzzles, or continuing education to keep their minds sharp.

- **Social Engagement:** They value staying connected with family, friends, and communities to nurture relationships and avoid isolation.
- **Purpose-Driven Living:** They often pursue meaningful goals, whether through volunteering, mentoring, creative pursuits, or exploring personal passions.
- **Health Awareness:** They take proactive steps to manage chronic conditions, maintain a healthy diet, and seek preventive care to optimize their well-being.
- **Adaptability:** They are resilient and open to change, embracing new technologies, lifestyles, or skills to stay connected and independent.

Is this you? It can be!

My goal is to provide you with information, specific exercises, stretches, and strategies to help you stay active and independent.

I am a baby boomer (born between 1946 – 1964). My generation has watched our parents age more quickly and become inactive once they retire.

We don't want that to happen to us!

More Baby Boomers are staying active by exercising their bodies, as well as their brains.

Do you aspire to be the man out riding his bike on a beautiful afternoon?

I am sure you don't want to be the man who needs a walker to get around. But good for you if you are using a walker and still get outside and walk.

Wouldn't you rather be the woman who goes to exercise class or swimming three days a week? It is much harder to be active when you need to have oxygen to survive.

Be an active ager!

You don't want to miss out on traveling because you can't walk up steps? Be fit to travel.

I work with my active agers to prepare them for traveling. We work on strengthening their legs to support the knees so they can walk up and down steps.

Do people have pain sometimes walking up and down stairs? Yes, I am one of them. However, the pain can be reduced by strengthening the muscles around your knees. I know everyone is different and deal with different aches and pains. Just do what you can to strengthen your body so you can be more active.

Do you want to be able to play with your grandchildren?

Can you play tennis or pickle ball with your friends?

Are you able to get down on the floor with your grandchildren?

Try new activities!

Be active together with your partner, it will bring more joy into your lives. Try kayaking, snow shoeing, hiking, or bike riding.

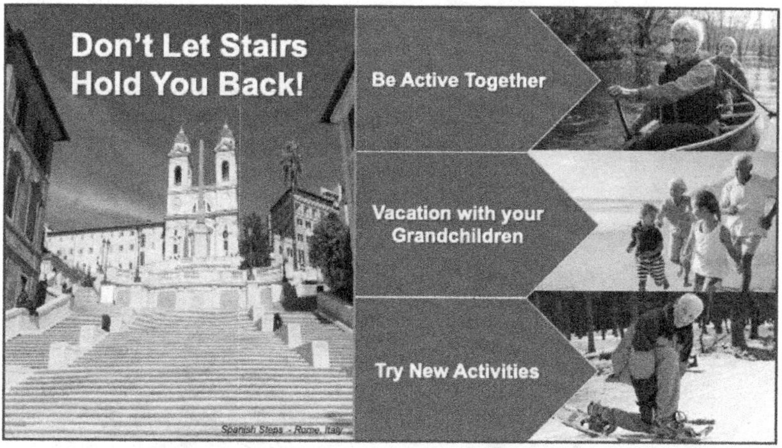
Don't Let Stairs
Hold You Back!
Be Active Together
Vacation with your Grandchildren
Try New Activities
Spanish Steps - Rome, Italy

At the time of writing this book, Dick Van Dyke is 99 years old and has a great attitude. He works out every day! He talked about why he exercised. It started out to look good in his 30's, then he wanted to stay fit in his 50's. Once he was in his 70's and 80's, he wanted to stay ambulatory and avoid going to assisted living. Dick Van Dyke is the prime example of "Exercise is the Fountain of Youth".

Lifestyle vs Genetics

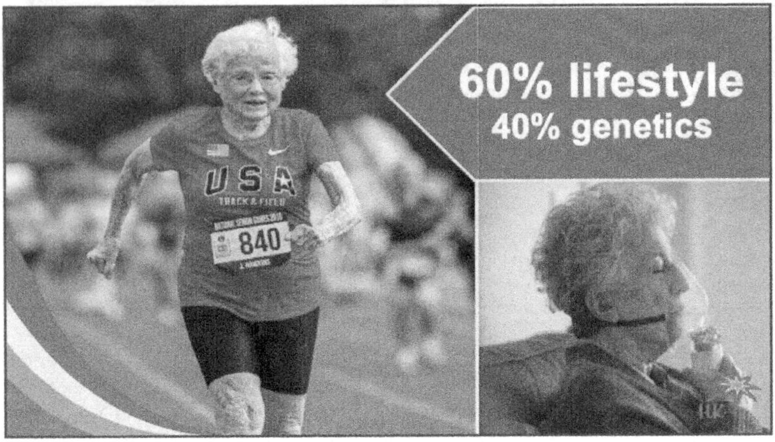

Your Health is 60 percent Lifestyle (or more) and 40 percent Genetics.

The woman running in this photo is Julia Hawkins, an American sprinter and cyclist who set the World Record in 2017 for the 100-meter dash in her age group (100-104).

The following are several studies that show you can add years to your life with lifestyle changes. The results are consistent in showing that certain lifestyle changes will add years to your life and life to your years.

In this first study, it shows how five healthy habits can extend your life by 12 – 14 years.

Harvard Study: Lifestyle and Life Expectancy

In this study (*Circulation* (2018), Harvard T.H. Chan School of Public Health) they followed 123,000 participants (Nurses' Health Study and Health Professionals Follow-Up Study)[1] for 30+ years. What they found was by adopting five healthy habits you could extend your life expectancy by **14 years longer for women and 12 years longer for men.**

The five factors in the study were:

1. Not smoking
2. Maintaining a healthy weight (BMI 18.5 – 24.9)
3. Eating a healthy diet (high in fruits, vegetables, whole grains, and low in processed foods)
4. Exercising regularly (>=30 minutes/day of moderate to vigorous activity).
5. Limiting alcohol consumption (<=1 drink/day for women, <=2 for men).

These habits reduced the risk of all-cause mortality by about seventy-four percent. All-cause mortality refers to the overall death rate from any cause, regardless of the specific reason for death.

This next study shows the areas in the world where people live the longest and some of the lifestyle habits they have in common.

Blue Zone Studies

Blue Zones are areas where people live longer than other areas of the world. Blue Zones are Okinawa, Japan;

Sardinia, Italy; Nicoya, Costa Rica; Ikaria, Greece; and Loma Linda, California.

The findings of this study, *Blue Zones Project* by *National Geographic Society* and Dan Buettner, were common lifestyle habits shared by the longest-living populations included:

- A plant-heavy diet
- Daily physical activity integrated into life (e.g., walking, gardening)
- Strong social connections and purpose in life.
- Stress reduction practices (e.g., naps, meditation).

The impact was life expectancy in these areas surpassed global averages by 8-12 years.

This next study was of interest to me since I am predisposed to Alzheimer's disease due to my mother's illness. It shows the six lifestyle factors that can add up to 14 years to your life.

MIND Diet and Alzheimer's Study

This study done by *Alzheimer's & Dementia* in 2015 followed over 900 participants aged 58-98 for an average of 4.5 years.[2]

What they found was:

- Adherence to the MIND diet (Mediterranean-DASH Intervention for Neurodegenerative Delay) reduced the risk of Alzheimer's by **53%** in strict followers and **35%** in moderate followers.
- Diet quality is linked to longevity and cognitive health in aging populations.

These studies and others consistently show that lifestyle changes—such as healthy eating, regular exercise, not smoking, and social engagement—can significantly increase life expectancy by **up to 10–14 years.**

This summary table of Lifestyle Factors & Longevity Impact makes it very clear what the cause and effect of each lifestyle factor can make on your life.

Lifestyle Factor	Impact on Longevity
Non-smoking	+10 years
Regular physical activity	+7–10 years
Healthy diet (e.g., plant-based)	+4–10 years
Moderate alcohol consumption	+4–5 years
Social connections	+5–10 years
Managing stress (e.g., meditation)	+3–5 years

These are strong reasons to make some lifestyle changes that will increase your longevity.

It is never too late to start making changes.

Here are some people who I am sure incorporated some of the healthy lifestyle habits in their life and did not let their age get in their way.

Julia "Hurricane" Hawkins (shown in the previous Lifestyle vs Genetics picture) was an extraordinary American athlete who began her sprinting career at the remarkable age of 100. Again, it is never too late to start!

Initially, Hawkins took up competitive cycling at age 75, participating in the National Senior Games and securing six gold medals in 5K and 10K cycling events. At 100 years old, her children encouraged her to transition to running. In 2017, at the USA Track and Field

Outdoors Masters Championships, she set a world record in the 100-meter dash for the 100–104 age category with a time of 39.62 seconds.

In 2021, at 105 years old, Hawkins became the first female athlete to record a time in the 100-meter dash within the 105+ age category, finishing in 1:02.95 at the Louisiana Senior Games. She was not the only one in her age category!

Julia Hawkins passed away on October 22, 2024, in Baton Rouge, at the age of 108. She was celebrated for her athletic achievements and as an inspiration for active aging, demonstrating that it's never too late to pursue new challenges.

Anne Lorimor (Mountaineer) became the oldest person to summit Mount Kilimanjaro, Africa's highest peak at age 89. Anne completed the climb to raise funds for children and to show that age is not a barrier to great achievements. She had first climbed Kilimanjaro at age 85 and beat her own record later at age 89.

George Jedenoff (Skier) started skiing at age 43 and continued skiing every year into his 100s. He credited his longevity to regular exercise, optimism, and enjoying life.

Fauja Singh (Marathon Runner) became the world's oldest marathon runner after completing his last full marathon at age 101. He began running marathons at age 89 and completed nine marathons.

Along with some of these high achievers' stories, I would like to share some stories from my clients.

One of my clients who took my classes went to Egypt with her daughter and kayaked down the Nile River. They went on a 3-day kayaking trip. She was 72 years old at the time.

Another client from my classes went zip lining in Costa Rica at the age of 76. She went hiking in Peru with her daughter at the age of 79. When she came back from their Peru trip, she said her daughter told her she had a hard time keeping up with her on the hikes.

Not every goal needs to be a huge goal. I had one client who was 82. His goal was to be able to climb up the bleachers with ease when he flew to California to see a tennis tournament. We worked hard together to make sure he could do just that. He went up and down the staircase in his home 10 times in a row each day to make sure he could do it. He came home from the tournament so excited because he just walked up those bleachers and sat himself down without any problems.

Another client, who has had both knees and both hips replaced and is in her eighties, goes hiking and camping every year. Last year she went on a safari with her grandchildren. They camped in tents the whole time. Nothing stops her!

A lot of the reason why these people accomplish their goals is their attitude. They have the attitude that they can do it, and they do it. Of course, there is a lot of prep work ahead of time to accomplish their goal.

Fitness is the Fountain of Youth! Anyone who knows me, knows that is my motto.

Stay active to stay young!

Key Points

- Your Health is 60 percent Lifestyle (or more) and 40 percent Genetics. More Baby Boomers are staying active by exercising their bodies, as well as their brains.
- Several studies show that changing some lifestyle habits can add many years to your life. Lifespan is the total number of years we live whereas, healthspan is how many of those years we remain healthy and free from disease.
- Julia Hawkins won the one-hundred-yard dash at age 105. She didn't start running until she was 100 years old!

2

Exercise

"Attending Holly's classes for over 10 years have helped to keep my heart muscle healthy. During my last stress test, the attendant was amazed at how fast and how long I could go for my age."

~ JOHN F

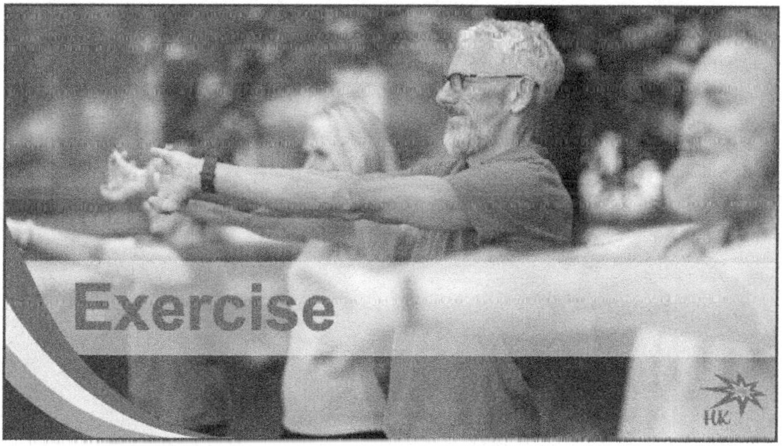

Exercise is very important to staying fit and healthy. But let's define the types of exercise we need to stay fit and healthy.

Movement vs Exercise

Movement is any *intentional* or *unintentional* effort to move your body; it should *not* feel like a "challenge" to your body or your mind. For example: Walking, hiking, dancing, easy swimming, etc.

An Exercise Workout is an *organized* session of moderate-to-intense physical activity usually lasting about 30 minutes or longer. For example: Strength training, cardio, stretching, going to an exercise class or working with a trainer on a specific program.

Do you exercise now?

I know that a lot of people don't like to exercise. However, you can affect your fitness level and health by doing more purposeful movement.

I want to teach you about your body's **Total Daily Energy Expenditure** (TDEE)[3]

This TDEE chart shows where your daily calorie expenditure is going. That is, how your body burns the calories you consume.

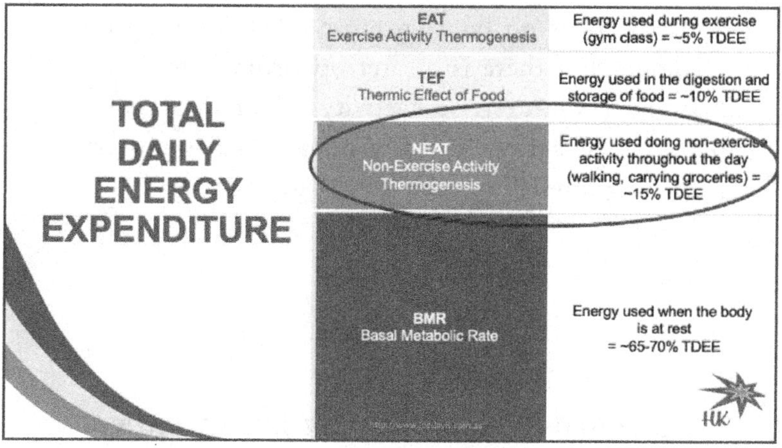

We start with your **BMR** (Basel Metabolic Rate). This is the energy your body uses when your body is at rest. Your BMR uses up about 65-70% of your TDEE. When your body is lying in bed and all your organs are functioning, this is how much energy your body uses.

Next is the **NEAT** (Non-Exercise Activity Thermogenesis) the energy used when you are doing non-exercise activity throughout the day – for example, walking or carrying groceries. NEAT uses about 15% of your TDEE.

The **TEF** (Thermic Effect of Food) is the energy used in the digestion and storage of the food we eat. The TEF uses about 10% of your TDEE. I will cover what foods to eat that have a high thermic effect in the Nutrition part of this book.

Then the **EAT** (Exercise Activity Thermogenesis) is the energy used during an exercise workout (a gym class or a structured workout). This uses about 5% of your TDEE.

Many focus on burning more calories during their workouts, but there is greater opportunity to increase NEAT (Non-exercise activity thermogenesis) in non-exercise activities like walking, carrying groceries, gardening, stretching, even fidgeting!

Here is the big TAKEAWAY:

NEAT
(or purposeful movement like walking)
is THE best way to
increase energy expenditure and
influence your overall health!

I want you to read the previous sentence again!

It is not the workout at the gym or the exercise class that will have the most effect on your Total Daily Energy Expenditure, it is the purposeful movement that you can do every day.

Now, the workout at the gym or the exercise class is important too, and I will get into those reasons soon, but for those of you who don't like to go to the gym, you are in control of increasing the **NEAT** (Non-Exercise Activity Thermogenesis) in your lifestyle.

When I talk about exercise being one of the pillars to staying fit, sharp, and independent, I am referring to three types of exercise:

1. Cardio Vascular Exercise
2. Strength Training
3. Flexibility

Cardio Vascular Exercise

Here are a few reasons to do cardio vascular exercise:

1. It enhances the hippocampus part of your brain. The hippocampus is where your memory is stored.
2. It helps keeps your heart and lungs healthy.
3. It can be a good social activity you can enjoy doing with family or friends.

I know that motivation to exercise can be a problem. I experience times when I am not motivated to exercise as well. There are ways to help you stay motivated.

Activity monitors are a great way to stay motivated. I am not going to get into which activity monitor is best. I had my client's using pedometers before the wrist band activity monitors came into play.

I find that if you are a competitive person, you like to see yourself accomplish your daily goal. I know I do. You could also enter in a challenge with other people. If you all use the same activity monitor, you can add each other as friends in the associated App and see each other's activity for the day.

The 10,000 steps a day recommendation came from the American Heart Association.

If you have a desk job, it is challenging to jump into getting 10,000 steps a day.

This is what I recommend for my clients:

- For the first **two weeks,** start with a goal of 4,000 steps per day during the work days, and 6,000 steps on non-work days. That may be a reach for some people. If you are in an office, make a habit of walking to the other side of the building to use the restroom. Take the stairs whenever possible or when you need a bit of a cardio break, walk up and down the stairs. Park farther from the building so you have to take more steps getting into the building and walking back to your car. For your safety, make sure it will be well lit if you are walking in or out in the dark.

- For the next two weeks (**weeks 3 & 4**), your goal is 6,000 steps per day during the work days and 8,000 steps on non-work days.
- The next two weeks (**weeks 5 & 6**), your goal is 8,000 steps per day during the work days and 10,000 steps on non-work days.
- Finally, **after 6 weeks** your goal is 10,000 steps per day on work days and maybe up it to 12,000 steps on non-work days.

This gives you a ramp up time to get to the 10,000 steps per day. For goal-oriented people this gives you daily achievements (short term goal) and a plan to achieve your long-term goal (10,000 steps per day). Achieving a goal daily is a huge motivator to continuing to work towards a long-term goal.

There are more accurate studies now that show 150 minutes a week of active cardio is beneficial. That could be 5 days of 30 minutes a day of active cardio.

Active cardio is not walking the dog unfortunately. The dog makes too many stops to smell and do their business for it to be active.

Music

Another thing that helps to motivate you is music. Put your favorite music on while you are working out and it becomes easier to do.

I used to run on the treadmill. I never really enjoyed running, but I did it because it helped me maintain a healthy weight. I would put music on that was 145 bpm (beats per minute), then I would run to the music like I was dancing. Sometime my arms would be flying around, just like I was dancing. I love to dance. The time flew by and it became a fun thing to do.

I have a client that has a hard time getting motivated to exercise when she gets home from work at night. I recommend she put on her favorite music and just dance around her living room. Now she does that to get some cardio in before she starts her strength training workout.

Whichever way motivates you the most to get out there and move, use it. I like goals so I still work towards the step goal. I teach exercise classes so I get my 150 minutes of active cardio in each week as well.

Strength Training

Here are a few reasons you want to do strength training:

1. Strength training is key to maintaining and building your muscles.
2. Adding muscle to your body will increase your metabolism so you burn more calories.
3. Strength training helps increase your bone density.

4. The stronger you are, the longer you will be able to live independently.

What is strength training?

Strength training is a type of exercise that involves using weights, resistance bands, machines, or body weight to build muscle strength and endurance.

Strength training is key to maintaining and building your muscles.

Everyone thinks that you lose muscle as you age. Here is the truth, you don't lose muscle because you are aging, you lose muscle because you stop being active with activities that were building your muscles.

Adding strength training, whether with dumbbells, resistance tubes/bands, exercise machines at the gym, or just your body weight, will help you in a number of ways.

The stronger you are the more you will be able to do your Activities of Daily Living which allows you to live independently longer.

Ideally, you want to do a strength training workout at least two times per week. Preferably three times per week.

I have my clients, which I will refer to them as Active Agers, **do 20 push-ups a day.** This increases their upper body strength.

Not everyone is going to drop down and give me 20!

There are many ways to do a push-up:

- Push-up against the wall (beginner)

- Push-up against the kitchen counter (beginner/intermediate)
- Push-up from a weight bench or chair (beginner/intermediate)
- Push-up on the floor on your knees. This is called a modified push-up, not a girly push-up! (beginner/intermediate)
- Push-up on the floor from your feet. (intermediate/advanced)
- Push-up on balance ball with feet on the ball (advanced)
- Push-up on balance ball with hands on a weighted medicine ball (advanced)
- Push-up using suspension straps, hands in the handles (intermediate/advanced)
- Push-up using suspension straps, feet in the handles (advanced)

There are still more ways to do a push-up then I have shown above. I filmed one episode on my TV show "Get Healthy with Holly" that was titled 20 ways to progress your push-up. As your strength grows, you want to progress on to more challenging push-ups.

Here are some of the benefits of strength training:

- More upper body strength to help you push yourself up from a fall.
- Increased strength should you need to defend yourself. The stronger you are the stronger your punch or push is.
- Your body definition improves. Your arms and body will look more toned. Don't worry, you won't

look like a body builder. They work a lot harder and longer on the strength training than 20 push-ups a day or by attending a strength training class.

- The more muscles you have around your joints, the more protection you have for them should you fall.

  I know from experience. I fell on black ice once and dislocated my shoulder. When I finally got up, I popped my shoulder back in place. The emergency room doctor said that the amount of muscle around my shoulder joint stopped the dislocation from being worse. The muscle didn't let my bone move very far.
- You will look good and feel good about the way you look in (and out) of your clothes.
- If you golf, a stronger back and core will help you hit the ball farther down the fairway. It won't help you to hit it straight down the fairway (you need some skill for that), but it will definitely help you to hit it farther.

  I worked with a client one day at 6am. He was going golfing that day so I gave him a workout that would help him have a great game. I said to him "You are going to have the best game ever today." He was skeptical. That night I received an email from him saying he played the best game he had ever played.
- If you have back pain or maybe a bulging disc, strengthening the Erector Spinae muscle will help to keep the bulging disc inside your spine and reduce sciatica pain. If your muscles are strong enough to keep the bulging disc from pushing on

your sciatic nerve, it reduces the pain and/or numbness you feel when the disc pushes on the nerve.

- If you live a sedentary lifestyle your Erector Spinae muscle does all the work to make up for weak abs, lats, and glutes. This causes undo stress on your back.

As we age, maintaining a healthy back is key to being able to stay active.

Sarcopenia

What is Sarcopenia? It is the loss of muscle mass, strength, and function in older adults.

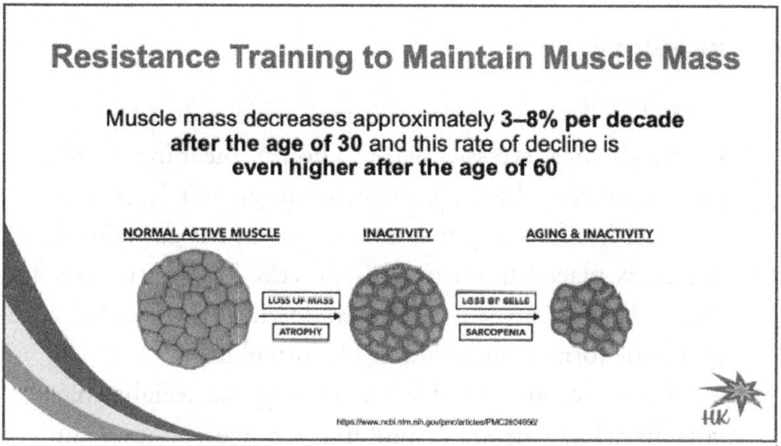

As you can see from the diagram[4] above, inactivity is a huge factor in muscle loss.

How does muscle loss Impact your Life?

Muscle loss:

- Increases your risk for falling, a leading cause of injury and death in older adults.

- Limits your mobility which can lead to loss of independence.
- Compromises your heart health *(your heart is a muscle)*.
- Restricts your metabolism, leading to weight gain and increased fat on your body.
- Increased risk of insulin resistance.
- Increased hospital complications.
- Additional complications for respiratory issues.
- Shortens life expectancy.

How exactly does strength training strengthen your bones?

Wolfe's Law

Wolfe's Law states that bone tissue will adapt to the mechanical stresses placed upon it, meaning it will grow stronger where it's subjected to greater force and remodel itself in response to changes in the functional demands placed upon it. This process is a continuous cycle of bone resorption (breakdown) by osteoclasts and bone formation (building) by osteoblasts.

This is accomplished by increasing the weight that you lift which assists in building stronger bones. Our bodies are in a constant state of bone remodeling. If you have more bone resorption than bone formation, you can end up with brittle bones or Osteoporosis. That is why it is important to continue strength training for the rest of your life.

I want to talk about how even if you do strength training regularly, after an injury and you go through the healing process, you will see that you have lost muscle mass (sarcopenia). I am a prime example of this. I had a bad fall on the ice years ago and tore my rotator cuff and my bicep tendon along with dislocating my shoulder. It required surgery to fix the tears. After surgery I did physical therapy. I, of course, did everything the physical therapist asked me to do. I have to set an example for my clients. We started with increasing my range of motion before moving onto improving strength. Prior to my fall, I was using 12lb weights while teaching my classes. It took me a year to build up my muscle strength to use 10lb weights while teaching class. It takes time to build muscle mass, it takes a lot less time to lose it. My recommendation is to start strength training if you are not already doing it and to continue for the rest of your life.

Flexibility

What is Flexibility? It is increasing the range of motion at joints by stretching muscles. Essentially it is making your body more flexible. Having your body be more flexible reduces your chance of injury.

Yoga, Pilates, and Tai Chi along with stretching are great ways to increase your flexibility. Tai Chi is also a great mind body exercise that is good for balance, as well as stress reduction.

It is important to keep our muscles strong, but it is also important to stretch them.

Having tight muscles can cause these common aches and pains:

- Tight hamstrings can cause lower back pain.
- Tight muscles in your arms can cause issues with your hands.
- Tight muscles on your neck can cause pain down your arm.
- Tight hips can cause pain in your back and legs.

Make sure to stretch the muscles that you use in your workouts. Don't shortchange the stretching; stretches will help reduce your soreness from exercise.

There are three common methods of stretching:

- **Static stretching:** Holding a stretch for a sustained period of time.
- **Dynamic stretching:** Moving through a range of motion with controlled movements.
- **Proprioceptive Neuromuscular Facilitation (PNF):** Utilizing muscle contractions to enhance stretching effectiveness.

Most people do static stretching. I find combining both static and dynamic stretches in my warm up routines to be very effective.

What benefits do we see from stretching:

- Improved athletic performance
- Reduced risk of injury
- Enhanced mobility and daily functioning
- Stress reduction
- Better posture

Look for opportunities to stretch your body. It is always better to warm up your muscles before stretching. Warm muscles stretch more and without injury.

If you are in a yoga class, please work within the limits of your body. Don't try to stretch as much as the person next to you. You have no idea how long they have been doing yoga and they may be more flexible than you.

I have a client who is a physician in the emergency room of a local hospital. He told me that they see more injured people in the emergency room from yoga classes than they do from down hill skiing (the hospital is close to a ski mountain). Work within the limits of your body. It is not a competition when you are in a yoga or stretch class.

These are the four stretches that my clients feel are the most important to them:

1. Yoga Cat/Cow stretch. You can do this stretch on the floor on all fours or standing leaning over with your hands above your knees. This stretch loosens up your lower back. If you are sitting for a long period of time, this stretch will help loosen your back and reduce pain.

Start in the tabletop position (on your hands and knees) on your mat. Round your back as you exhale, then extend your back as you inhale. If you are standing, lean forward a bit and place your hands on your legs above your knees. Round your back as you exhale, then extend your back as you inhale.

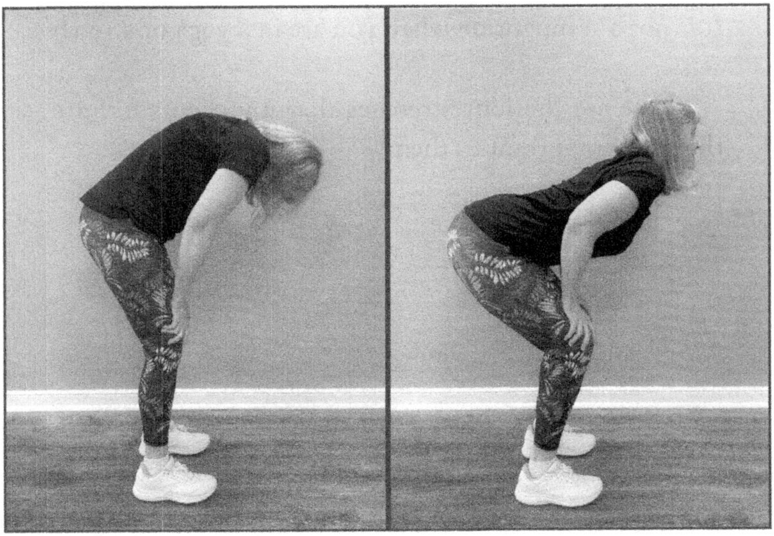

2. Seated Piriformis Stretch. The piriformis is a small, pear-shaped muscle located deep in your buttock, behind the gluteus maximus. It runs diagonally from the lower spine to the outer hip. When the piriformis becomes tight, shortened, or inflamed, it can irritate or compress the sciatic nerve, which runs just beneath it.

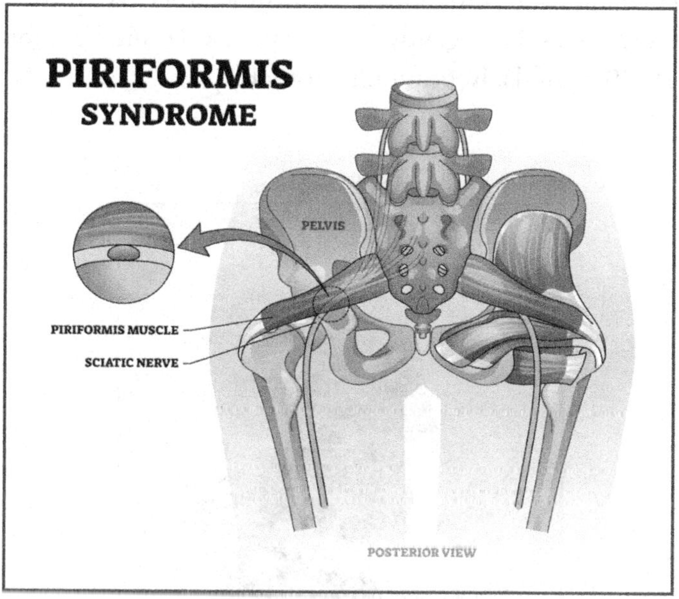

This is a very common cause for Sciatic pain or tingling.

Piriformis stretches are often prescribed for people with:

- Sciatica
- Sacroiliac joint dysfunction
- Chronic low back pain
- Postural imbalances from prolonged sitting

You perform this stretch from a seated position on a chair, place one foot on top of the other knee. With your hand, press down gently on your bent knee and hold for 10-20 seconds. Repeat on the other leg.

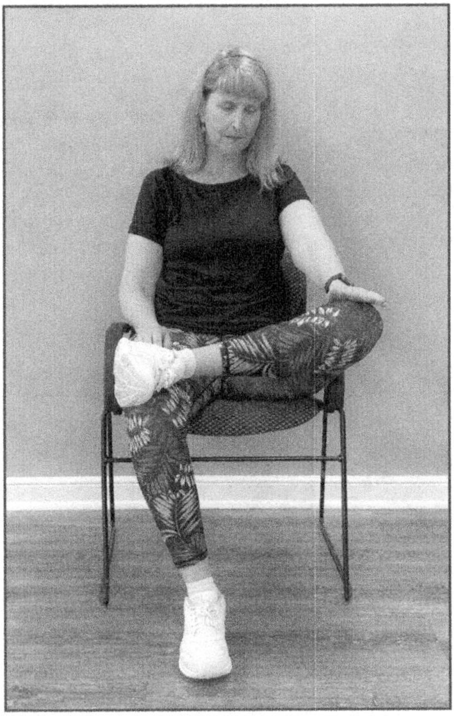

3. Standing Straight Arm Neck Rotation Stretch. This stretch is important to do to help when you drive. It helps you to stretch your neck so you are able to look both ways when you are turning in your car. One of my Active Agers in class loves this stretch because she said when she was driving with her father, he couldn't turn his head far enough to see both ways. She remembered how scary it was because he would pull out and not know if a car was coming.

In a standing position, bring one arm out in front of you, as you move that arm to the side, turn you head in the opposite position. Try to look behind you with your eyes. Hold for 10-20 seconds. Repeat on the other arm.

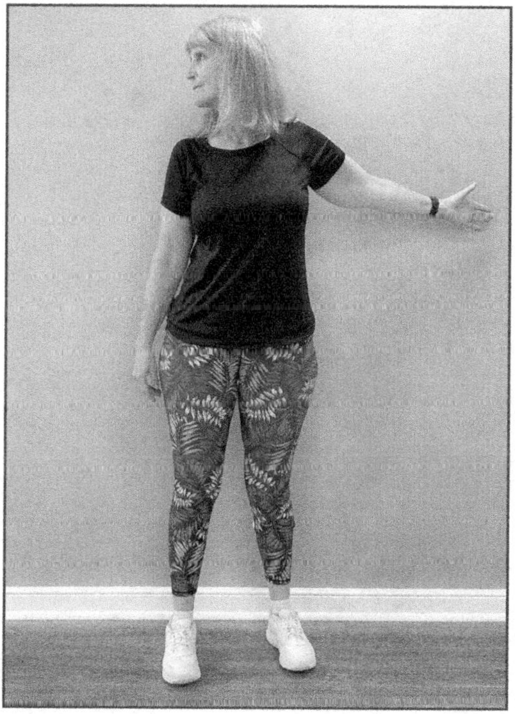

4. Standing Calf and Triceps Stretch. This stretch is not just a stretch, but it is also a balance exercise.

In a standing position, move one foot on the ground behind you. Make sure your heel is on the ground. Tighten your core for balance. Move the arm on the same side of your body up and bend at the elbow (your hand coming down towards your back). Place your other hand on the elbow and gently press it up towards the sky. Hold for 10-20 seconds. Repeat on the other side.

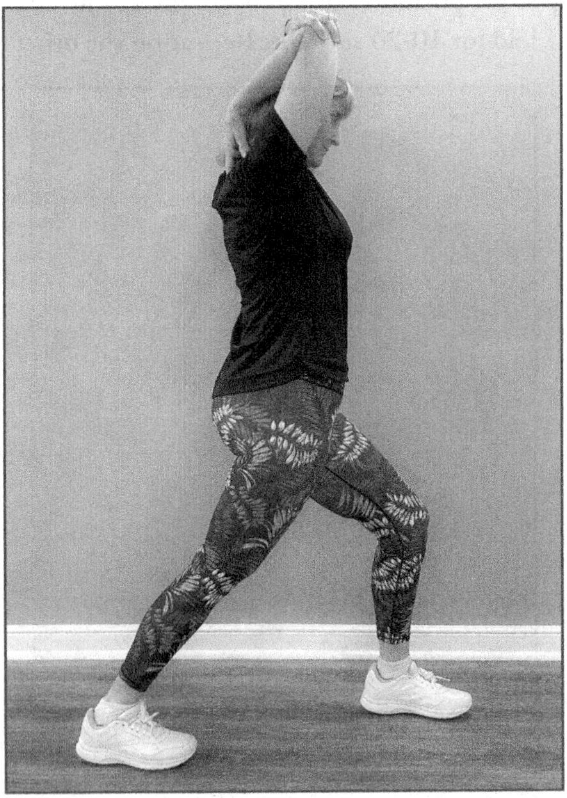

Motion is Lotion

This is something I am always saying in my classes and to my clients. It is true.

In that same fall that I wrote about earlier, I also ended up with back problems.

I know now that I need to go for a walk every day, as well as do my strengthening exercises to help stave off back pain.

The last thing you should do when you have a stiff back or pain is to sit or lie down all day. It may take a little bit to get started, but once you get started you realize how much you need to keep moving.

One of my clients told me she had back spasms in the past and tried to just lie down and rest but got no relief. She decided she was just going to get up and go about her day and found out that within a few hours she was doing yard work without pain. She told me before taking my class she had never heard the saying "Motion is Lotion".

Key Points

- Keep moving! Staying active in your daily activities, using **NEAT** (Non-Exercise Activity Thermogenesis) will burn more calories. The best exercise is walking. Get outside and move!
- If you can't go outside to walk, walk around your house. Just Walk!
- Add strength training 2-3 times per week to avoid sarcopenia and to increase your muscle mass. Stretching helps to reduce soreness and can reduce pain caused by tight muscles. Do 20 push-ups a day.
- Exercise with a buddy, it keeps you motivated. **Motion is Lotion!** Exercise helps reduce aches and pains.

After each pillar you will get a few questions to help you come up with your **Personal Thrive Formula.**

My goal is for you to have a formula for you to thrive by the time you finish reading this book. The questions in each section will help you look at your current lifestyle and see where you can make some changes and add healthy habits to your lifestyle.

Take a few moments to analyze what you are doing now versus what you could be doing to continue thriving as you age.

Personal Thrive Formula Exercise – A body in motion, stays in motion!

Answer the questions below as it relates to exercise:

Check the one that applies to you.

Currently, exercise for me is:

- ❑ High priority
- ❑ Somewhat of a priority
- ❑ Not a priority

How would you describe your current mindset towards exercise?

- ❑ It feels like a chore
- ❑ I'm consistent
- ❑ I can't live without it!

Fitness/Exercise I enjoy or enjoyed in the past includes:

____

____

What are you doing right now to build bone density and muscle?

____

____

Lifestyle changes as it relates to exercise:

1. How will you add more purposeful movement into your daily life:

1. ____

2. ____

3. ____

2. Improve bone density with these daily steps

1. ____

2. ____

3. ____

How will you add in Resistance Training?

____

____

What time of day will you exercise?

____

____

Will you move or exercise with a friend? (Having a workout or walking partner helps you be accountable.)

____

____

Determine the type of movement you enjoy and do it!

Put exercise/movement in your calendar!

"I have had the pleasure of working with Holly for the last five years. Her exercise and nutrition programs have helped me stay more active, healthy and helped me keep up with my grandchildren.

Holly's counseling on how to incorporate daily movement with simple steps on improving my daily nutrition, have improved my overall health and well-being. I am also grateful to Holly for guiding me into a healthier mindset and relationship with food.

Thank you, Holly!"

~MARY R.

3

Nutrition

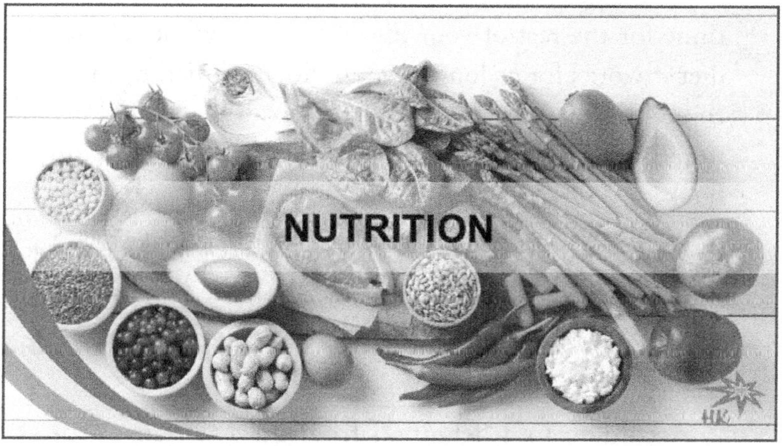

What do you think of when I say Nutrition?

Do you think of eating a vegetarian diet (no meat, poultry, or fish)? Maybe a Vegan diet (no dairy, meat, eggs, or honey)?

Do you think of eating your fruits and veggies?

According to the Merriam-Webster dictionary, **nutrition** is the act or process of nourishing or being nourished. It is the foods you eat to nourish your body.

There are so many diets circulating around, along with many theories on how to eat, when to eat, and when to fast, that it gets overwhelming. What I will tell you is, do what works for you. It may be a combination of different diets, timing on when to eat, as well as how long you should fast. Do what makes sense for you!

I want you to learn to eat in a way that you can continue for the rest of your life. When you go on a strict diet it works for as long as you follow the diet. But is it something you can follow for the rest of your life? Portion control is key and I will be addressing it later in the book.

Before we get into what foods you should eat, let's talk about how often you should eat and why.

Metabolism

According to a definition from the Merriam-Webster dictionary, **metabolism** is the sum of the processes by which a particular substance is handled in the living body. Basically, metabolism is the rate with which your body burns fuel.

When and why does your metabolism slow down?

Age isn't really the factor in why it slows down, although most people see the slow-down in their 40's and 50's. The real reason is the loss of muscle mass and leading a less active life.

There are ways to speed up your metabolism. I have been speaking about the ways to increase your metabolism for the past 20 plus years.

The more muscle you have on your body, the faster your metabolism.

You can use the Thermic Effect of Food (TEF) to your advantage.

For our purposes in this book, let's think about your metabolism as a fire in the fireplace.

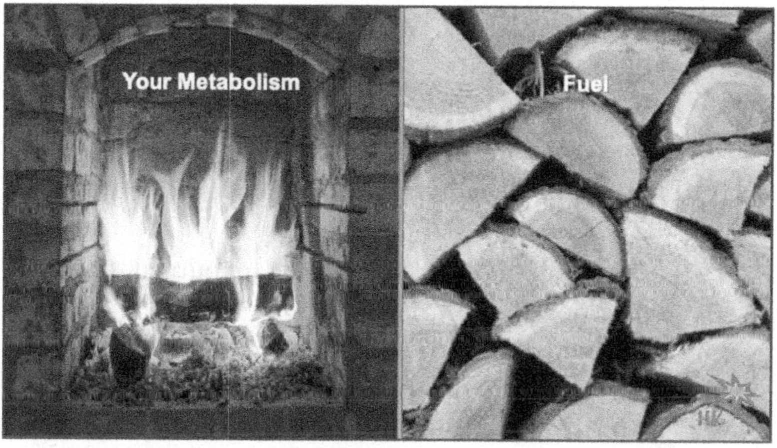

Let's pretend you heat your home with fire (fireplace or woodstove). The first thing you do in the morning is put some logs on the fire to get the fire burning hot. Then a few hours later you put more logs on the fire to keep it burning at a higher rate. If you go too long between putting logs on the fire, the fire dies down. It is better to feed the fire logs at a consistent rate (every few hours) over the day to keep it burning at the optimal rate for heating your home.

Think of your metabolism like the fire in your fire place. When you get up in the morning, you want to feed it breakfast so it can start burning at a higher rate (somewhere between waking and 1-1½ hours after waking up). Then in order to keep your metabolism burning at a consistent rate all day long, you need to eat every 3-3½ hours. It is just like putting the logs in the fireplace.

The higher the metabolism, the more calories you burn. The goal is to eat small meals 5-6 times a day. These are not big meals. Some meals may be a simple snack like ¼ cup of nuts or a low-fat cheese stick.

You want these meals or foods to have a higher thermic effect.

Protein has the highest thermic effect on your body.

Here are the Thermic Effect of Food (TEF) values for the different types of foods:

- **Protein**: 20-30% of its calories are burned during digestion
- **Carbohydrates**: 5-10% of its calories are burned during digestion
- **Fats**: 0-3% of its calories are burned during digestion

What does this mean? This means that if you eat 100 calories from protein, around 20-30 calories are burned just for digestion and metabolism.

Here is where you let the thermic effect of food work for you to either lose weight or to maintain a healthy weight.

It is best to eat a supportive meals 5-6 times a day.

> "A supportive meal is one which provides material from which we can build and maintain cells, one which allows us to maintain a balance of hormone production allowing for ongoing fat release, as well as one which provides adequate 'highly thermic' fuel for energy production. While fat, for example, requires very little work for digestion, a "supportive meal" is one which in itself would ask the body to expend energy and produce heat at high levels."[5]

A "Supportive Meal" consists of:

- Lean Proteins
- Starchy Carbohydrates
- Fibrous Carbohydrates

Protein

What is a protein food? A protein food is any food that provides a significant amount of protein, an essential nutrient your body needs for building and repairing tissues, for making enzymes and hormones, and supporting overall health.

Put simply:

- Your body works hard to digest protein.

- Protein helps build and repair cells, muscles, bones, cartilage, skin, and blood.
- Protein can help speed up your metabolism.
- Protein helps with weight loss because it helps you feel fuller.
- Protein helps improve your body composition.
- Protein can help balance blood glucose levels.
- Protein is important for growth and development for children, teens, and pregnant women.

HERE ARE EXAMPLES OF HEALTHY PROTEINS:	
Egg Whites	Fish (including shellfish)
Chicken Breast	Fat-free Dairy Products
Turkey Breast	Beans—cooked
Tofu (soy)	(black beans, kidney, chickpeas or lentils)

Starchy Carbohydrates

What are starchy carbohydrates? Starchy carbohydrates are a type of carbohydrate that contain a high amount of starch, a complex carbohydrate that provides the body with energy. These foods are digested more slowly than simple sugars, leading to a more gradual release of glucose into the bloodstream.

You do not want to eliminate carbohydrates from your diet.

Your brain relies on carbohydrates as its primary source of energy. When you eat carbs, they break down into glucose, which fuels brain cells for consistent energy, mental clarity, and mood stability.

This is why when people eat a high protein, low carb diet, their brain feels fuzzy and it is hard for them to concentrate. Their brain is not getting what it needs to function optimally.

There are good choices for starchy carbs and bad choices for starchy carbs. Stay away from the sugary starchy carbs like cereal, cookies, and processed foods. The added sugar is not good for you.

HERE ARE EXAMPLES OF HEALTHY STARCHY CARBOHYDRATES:		
Barley	Lima Beans	Red Beans
Corn	Black-Eyed Peas	Lentils
Oatmeal	Whole-Wheat Flour	Popcorn
Tomatoes	Pasta	Yams/Sweet Potato
Peas	Rice (Brown Jasmine, Basmati)	Shredded Wheat
Potatoes	Butternut Squash	Cream of Rice
Cereal (low sugar)	Couscous	Corn Tortillas

Fibrous Carbohydrates

Fibrous Carbohydrates are complex carbohydrates that are rich in fiber, a type of indigestible carbohydrate that plays a crucial role in digestion and overall health. Fibrous Carbs have the following benefits:

- Help to clean out your digestive tract.
- Good for weight loss as it moves slowly through the body which makes you feel fuller longer.
- Does not spike your blood sugar level.

- The fiber can help reduce heart disease by preventing your body from absorbing fat and cholesterol.
- They are high in nutrients like vitamins and minerals.

HERE ARE EXAMPLES OF HEALTHY FIBROUS CARBOHYDRATES:		
Asparagus	Artichoke	Broccoli
Kale	Brussel Sprouts	Cabbage
Cauliflower	Carrots	Celery
Cucumber	Eggplant	Green Beans
Green Peppers	Mushrooms	Yellow Peppers
Red Peppers	Okra	Onion
Pumpkin	Spinach	Zucchini

Fresh vegetables and fruit are best, but frozen veggies and fruits are usually frozen right when they come off the field so they are just as good.

MIND Diet (Mediterranean-DASH Intervention for Neurodegenerative Delay)

I would be remiss if I didn't speak about the MIND Diet since I promote and teach brain health.

Most doctors like the **MIND Diet** because it combines the brain-health benefits of the **Mediterranean Diet** and the **DASH Diet** (Dietary Approaches to Stop Hypertension). It specifically targets brain health and has shown promise in reducing the risk of Alzheimer's disease and promoting overall cognitive function.

Here are a few reasons why the MIND Diet is highly regarded:

1. **Evidence-Based Benefits for Brain Health**
   - Cognitive Decline Prevention: Studies suggest that the MIND Diet can reduce the risk of Alzheimer's by up to 53% in those who adhere to it strictly and by 35% even in moderate followers.
   - Neuroprotection: The diet emphasizes foods rich in antioxidants, healthy fats, and anti-inflammatory properties, which help protect the brain from oxidative stress and inflammation—two key factors in cognitive decline.
2. **Combination of Two Proven Diets**
   - The MIND Diet incorporates the heart-healthy principles of the Mediterranean and DASH diets, which are both well-supported by research for reducing risks of cardiovascular disease, hypertension, and stroke—all of which are linked to brain health.
3. **Simple and Flexible**
   - The diet is not overly restrictive. It focuses on increasing the intake of 10 brain-healthy food groups (like leafy greens, berries, nuts, whole grains, and fish) while reducing 5 unhealthy groups (like red meats, butter, cheese, sweets, and fried foods).
   - The approach is more about adding healthy foods than cutting out everything, making it easier for people to adhere to over the long term.

4. **Whole-Body Health**
   - Since what's good for the brain is also generally good for the heart, the MIND Diet contributes to overall health by improving vascular function, reducing inflammation, and lowering the risk of chronic diseases.
5. **Practical for Older Adults**
   - Doctors working with aging populations appreciate that the MIND Diet is nutrient-dense yet accessible. It includes foods that are widely available and generally affordable, which is important for older adults who might be on fixed incomes.
6. **Supportive of Aging Actively**
   - For those looking to age actively and maintain independence longer, the diet's support for mental clarity, memory, and physical health aligns well with your goals of healthy aging.

Integrating the MIND Diet into your lifestyle to promote active aging involves more than just changing what's on your plate—it's about creating habits that support both physical and mental vitality.

Start to build your meals around Brain-Healthy foods.

The MIND Diet emphasizes 10 brain-healthy foods:

- **Leafy Greens:** Spinach, kale, and Swiss chard (Aim for 6+ servings per week)
- **Other Vegetables:** A variety of colors and types (At least 1 serving per day)
- **Berries:** Especially blueberries and strawberries (2+ servings per week)

- **Nuts:** Almonds, walnuts, pistachios (5 servings per week)
- **Whole Grains:** Oats, quinoa, brown rice (3 servings per day)
- **Fish:** Especially fatty fish like salmon (1+ serving per week)
- **Poultry:** Chicken or turkey (2 times per week)
- **Beans:** Lentils, chickpeas, and other legumes (4 times per week)
- **Olive Oil:** As your primary cooking oil
- **Wine (Optional):** Up to 1 glass per day (if approved by your doctor)

Doctors recommending the MIND diet say you should also pair your nutrition with Cognitive Engagement.

- **Cook Mindfully:** Experiment with new recipes to challenge your brain.
- **Learn While You Eat:** Try themed dinners with cultural or historical learning components.
- **Garden if You Can:** Growing your own vegetables adds physical activity and mental stimulation.

  My husband used to tend a large garden in the summer which produced more than we could eat. The past few years he had some big projects to do over the summer so instead we participated in a Consumer Supported Agriculture (CSA) program at a small farm in our town. CSA's offer the public a new way to invest in local agriculture, while enjoying delicious, fresh food throughout the season. Some weeks there would be vegetables that I had never tasted before and I would need to get creative with recipes including those foods. It was a nice mental challenge, as well as trying new foods.

Move with Purpose

Of course, physical activity complements the MIND Diet's brain-boosting benefits. The focus is on:

- **Regular Exercise:** Aim for 150 minutes of moderate-intensity cardio activity per week.
- **Incorporating Strength Training:** Maintains muscle mass and improves balance.
- **Combine Movement with Socialization:** Join a walking group, a dance class, or an exercise class.

It is also recommended to **Stay Socially Active**.

- Share Meals with Others: It promotes mental well-being and combats loneliness.
- Join Cooking Classes: Especially those focused on healthy, MIND Diet-friendly recipes.
- Engage in Community Activities: Potlucks, book clubs, or volunteer events.

I play Mahjong with a group of ladies every week. Not only is it social, it is good for my brain.

Make the changes Manageable.

- **Meal Prep:** Prepare brain-healthy meals in advance to avoid eating what is easy and convenient.

- **Set Small Goals:** Try adding one extra serving of vegetables daily or swap a sugary snack for nuts.
- **Adapt for Convenience:** Frozen berries and vegetables are just as healthy as fresh and often easier to keep on hand.

Put your Focus on Routine, Not Restrictions.

- **Morning Routine:** Start with a whole-grain breakfast (e.g., oatmeal with berries and nuts).
- **Balanced Snacks:** Keep nuts, seeds, and fresh fruits handy.
- **Flexible Dinners:** Swap out red meats for poultry or fish when possible.

Track Your Progress

- **Journaling:** Note how your mood, energy, and memory improve.

Holly's Helpful Hint

If weight loss is a goal, I always say "When you Log it, You Lose it". Logging your food intake helps you to lose weight because you have a better understanding of what you actually eat during the day.

Celebrate Wins: Whether it's trying a new recipe or sticking to your meal plan for a week. Do something to celebrate it.

I had one client in my weight loss clinic when she lost weight that week, she treated herself to a manicure. I used to hand out stickers when you lost weight in my weight loss clinics (don't underestimate the value of getting a sticker). One woman said she tried hard to make sure she got a sticker because when she went home from the clinic her little girl asked if she got a sticker and she did not want to disappoint her daughter.

Buy yourself flowers so that every time you look at them you feel your accomplishment all over again.

I created a Happy Dance for my "Fitness with Holly" class. Since I ask my clients to do 20 push-ups a day, when I ask in class who has done their push-ups, we celebrate those who did with a Happy Dance.

In my "Fusion Fitness" class, we email each other every day when we do our push-ups. Then we celebrate doing our push-ups with a pot luck dinner every quarter at different people's homes. The class is much smaller than my "Fitness with Holly" class and we are usually able to fit everyone around a large dining room table.

Many people need to see an example of the foods to eat in a particular diet. It gives them a better idea of whether they can be successful with the diet or not.

To help you out with what to eat on the MIND diet, here is a sample one-week meal plan :

MIND Diet One Week Meal Plan[6]

Monday

- **Breakfast:** Greek yogurt with raspberries and sliced almonds
- **Lunch:** Mediterranean salad with olive oil-based dressing, grilled chicken, whole wheat pita
- **Dinner:** burrito bowl with brown rice, black beans, fajita vegetables, grilled chicken, salsa, and guacamole

Tuesday

- **Breakfast:** whole wheat toast with almond butter, scrambled eggs
- **Lunch:** grilled chicken sandwich, blackberries, carrots
- **Dinner:** grilled salmon, side salad with olive oil-based dressing, brown rice

Wednesday

- **Breakfast:** steel-cut oatmeal with strawberries, hard-boiled eggs
- **Lunch:** Mexican-style salad with mixed greens, black beans, red onion, corn, grilled chicken, and olive oil-based dressing
- **Dinner:** chicken and vegetable stir-fry, brown rice

Thursday

- **Breakfast:** Greek yogurt with peanut butter and banana
- **Lunch:** baked trout, collard greens, black-eyed peas
- **Dinner:** whole wheat spaghetti with turkey meatballs and marinara sauce, side salad with olive oil-based dressing

Friday

- **Breakfast:** whole wheat toast with avocado, omelet with peppers and onions
- **Lunch:** chili made with ground turkey
- **Dinner:** Greek-seasoned baked chicken, oven-roasted potatoes, side salad, whole wheat dinner roll

Saturday

- **Breakfast:** overnight oats with strawberries and almond butter
- **Lunch:** fish tacos on whole wheat tortillas, brown rice, coleslaw, and pinto beans
- **Dinner:** chicken gyro on whole wheat pita, cucumber and tomato salad

Sunday

- **Breakfast:** spinach frittata, sliced apple with peanut butter
- **Lunch:** tuna salad sandwich on whole wheat bread, plus carrots and celery with hummus
- **Dinner:** curry chicken, brown rice, lentils, and a side salad

Keep in mind when putting dressing on your salad; most salad dressings you find at the store are not made primarily with olive oil, but you can easily make your own salad dressing at home.

To make a simple balsamic vinaigrette, combine 3 parts extra-virgin olive oil with 1-part balsamic vinegar. Add a little Dijon mustard, salt, and pepper and mix well.

Portion Control

We do need to talk about portion control. Most Americans eat more than the portion size of foods. When I was focused on helping people lose hundreds of pounds, I had my clients use a portion control plate to see what a proper portion size was. There are many varieties of portion control plates and containers to help you with portion size.

Here are some of my tips for portion control:

- If you are using a portion control plate. Once you put the appropriate portion size of food on the plate, transfer the food to your plate at home. This way you see what a proper portion size is on your plates. If your dinner plates are really big, get smaller plates because true portions will look small on your big plates. You can also eat from a luncheon plate.
- Be mindful of portion sizes. You may need to weigh food in the beginning before you can really judge the correct portion size of a food.
- Cheese is a tough one to get the portion size correct. I use this picture and in my live talks, I use the props for people to visual what 1oz, 3oz, or a head of cheese looks like. Yes, I put the cheese head on during my presentation. (I visited my brother in Wisconsin and went to Lambeau field, the Green Bay Packers stadium, where I bought the cheese head for my portion control demonstration.)
- Alcohol is another area where people may consume more than one portion without realizing it.

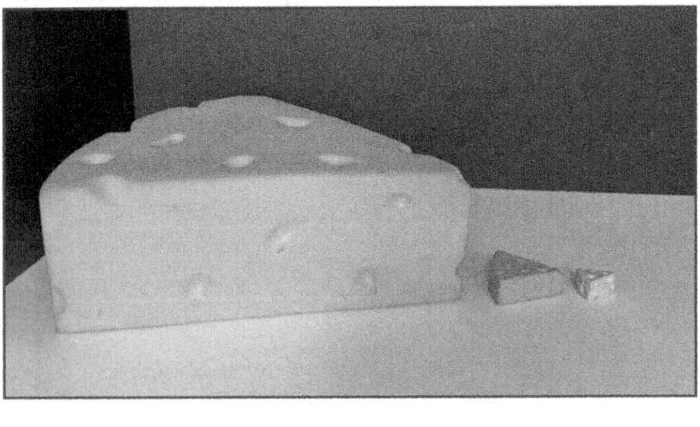

Understand the Standard Drink Sizes Across Different Types of Alcohol.

To drink mindfully, especially when focusing on active aging and your health, it's important to know what constitutes a standard drink. Each standard drink contains approximately 14 grams (0.6 ounces) of pure alcohol, regardless of the type of beverage.

Alcohol Type	Standard Drink Size	Average Alcohol by Volume (ABV)
Beer	12 ounces (355 ml)	~5% ABV
Craft or Strong Beer	8-10 ounces (237-296 ml)	~7-9% ABV
Wine	5 ounces (148 ml)	~12% ABV
Fortified Wine	3-4 ounces (89-118 ml)	~17-20% ABV
Liquor (Spirits) 80-proof	1.5 ounces (44 ml)	~40% ABV
Liqueurs/Cordials	2-3 ounces (59-89 ml)	~20% ABV
High-ABV Cocktails	Varies standard drink is ~1.5 oz of hard liquor	~40% ABV

Beer:

- **Pint:** *Caution:* A 16-ounce pint of beer is 1.3 standard drinks if the beer is 5% ABV.
- **High-ABV Beers:** For beers 8% ABV or higher, a 10-ounce pour may already be 1.5 - 2 standard drinks.

Wine:

- Use a measuring cup to understand what 5 ounces looks like in your glass.
- Wine glasses vary greatly, so avoid filling large goblets fully.

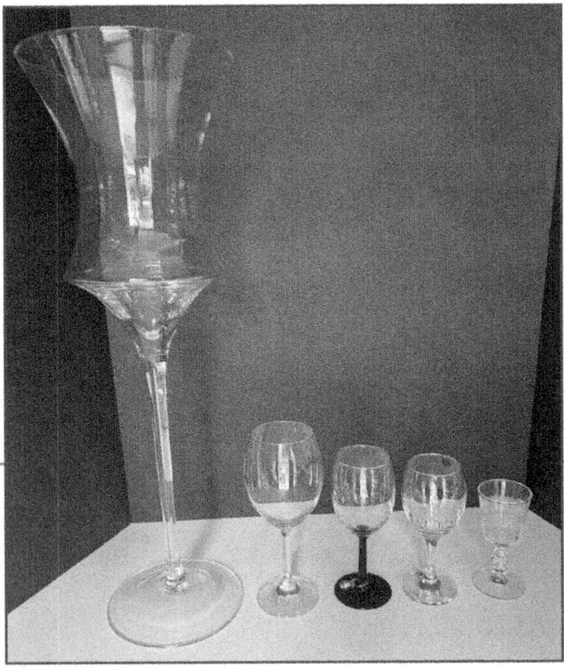

Holly's Helpful Hint

I recommend using a smaller glass with a proper portion. It will make the class look fuller. The smaller the glass the fuller it looks. Don't use the biggest glass!

Spirits & Cocktails:

- Measure 1.5 ounces using a jigger or shot glass.
- Be mindful of cocktails, as they may contain multiple types of alcohol, increasing the drink calorie count quickly.

Holly's Helpful Hint

For every class of alcohol have a glass of water. Alcohol dehydrates you. Dehydration is part of a hangover. If you drink a glass of water for every glass of alcohol you stay hydrated and have less hangover effects the next day.

Hydration

Hydration becomes increasingly critical as we age, and yet it's often overlooked. Seniors are particularly vulnerable to dehydration for a variety of reasons, and the consequences can be serious.

Why is hydration so important for Seniors:

- As we age, our thirst naturally decreases. You may not feel thirsty, even when your body is low on fluids.
- Our kidneys become less efficient at conserving water, which means the body loses fluids more easily and needs more replenishment.
- Many common medications for older adults—such as diuretics, blood pressure meds, and laxatives—increase fluid loss.
- Some seniors may struggle to access water due to limited mobility, memory issues, or even depression, making it harder to stay hydrated.
- Older adults have less lean body mass, which holds less water. That means they have a smaller "hydration reserve" to pull from.

There are many health benefits to staying hydrated. Staying hydrated helps:

- Maintains body temperature regulation
- Support brain function and alertness
- Keep joints lubricated and muscles functioning
- Aid in digestion and prevents constipation
- Helps your kidneys flush out toxins
- Supports heart health and circulation

I realize it is sometimes a challenge to drink enough water during the day. You should drink 6-8 cups of water each day.

Symptoms of dehydration can also be mistaken for symptoms of other ailments or diseases. Below are a few examples.

Dehydration Symptom	Could Be Mistaken For
Fatigue or weakness	Depression, anemia
Confusion or irritability	Dementia, UTI, stroke
Dizziness or lightheadedness	Low blood pressure, vertigo
Dry mouth or sunken eyes	Side effects of medication
Constipation	Poor diet, IBS
Rapid heart rate	Anxiety, cardiac issues
Low blood pressure	Heart issues, medication side effects

Here are some tips on how to drink more water:

- Drink 3-4 glasses of water before 12 noon. You don't want to drink too much water after dinner or you may need to go to the bathroom often during the night.
- Keep water easily accessible. Take your water bottle with you everywhere you go.
- Use hydration reminders (alarms, notes, or apps).
- Track when you drink water. Keep a tally during the day.
- Incorporate fluids through soups, fruits (watermelon), and herbal teas.
- Make water more appealing with infused flavors (like lemon or cucumber).

Hydration is a cornerstone of aging well—it impacts cognition, mobility, heart health, and overall vitality.

Drink more water!

Key Points

- When it comes to what diet to follow, do what works for you. It may be a combination of different diets, timing on when to eat, as well as how long you should fast. Do what makes sense for you!
- Use the thermic effect of food (TEF) as much as possible. Watch your portion sizes to maintain a healthy weight. The MIND diet doesn't focus on food alone. It is recommended to socialize, exercise, log your food (if weight loss is a goal), and get creative with your cooking.
- Go easy on the alcohol and stay hydrated! Drink 6-8 glasses of water per day.

Personal Thrive Formula Nutrition: Food as Fuel!

Answer the questions below as it relates to nutrition:

How familiar are you with sources of quality protein?

- ❑ Very familiar
- ❑ Somewhat familiar
- ❑ Not very familiar

Currently, would you say:

- ❑ I have not made it a priority to ensure I'm eating enough protein.
- ❑ I go through phases: sometimes I make eating enough protein a priority, other times it's a challenge
- ❑ Eating enough protein is a priority for me.

Currently, would you say:

- ❑ I have not made it a priority to ensure I'm eating enough vegetables/fruit.
- ❑ I go through phases: sometimes I make eating enough vegetables/fruit a priority, other times it's a challenge
- ❑ Eating enough vegetables and fruit is a priority for me.

Lifestyle changes as it relates to nutrition:

How will I incorporate protein, vegetables and fruit into my diet?

1. ______________________________

2. ______________________________

3. ______________________________

4. ______________________________

What is my strategy to drink more water each day?

____

____

Meal planning can make eating healthy easier.

4

Brain & Balance

"I have integrated the various exercises into my routine at my fitness center AND added Sudoku to my daily Wordle and Connections routine!

I really felt your course was helpful in improving my balance...AND brain!"

– JEANNE L

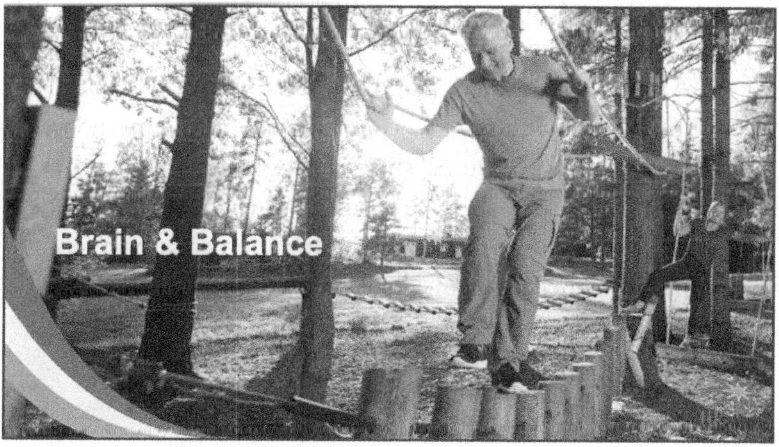

You start to lose your sense of balance earlier than you realize. It maintains a steady decline after age 50[7]. If you don't try to maintain your balance through balance activities, you lose your balance abilities. This is why as a senior, you are more susceptible to falls.

As I mentioned earlier, I have been teaching my Brains & Balance class for over 10 years. We spend half the class doing balance exercises (which include core and leg strength) and the other half of the class doing Brain Drills.

The premise of the class is when you increase your balance, you increase your cognitive abilities and when you increase your cognitive abilities, you increase your balance.

The following studies show there is a direct correlation that improving your balance also improves your cognition.

A study by Rogge et al. (2017)[8] demonstrated that a 12-week balance training program significantly improved memory and spatial cognition in healthy adults, suggesting that improving your balance can positively impact cognitive function.

A study by Doumas, Rapp, and Krampe et al. (2008)[9] found that older adults who practiced working memory training for 10 sessions showed improved balance by allocating more cognitive resources to the task, demonstrating that enhancing cognitive function can positively impact balance control; this suggests a link between cognitive improvement and better balance capabilities.

Balance

Why is balance so important? Good balance is crucial for everyday activities like walking, running, or even standing still. It helps prevent falls and injuries, especially as we age.

Falls are a leading cause of hospitalization and long-term care in the US. One fall can change your life forever.

I can attest to that. The fall I referred to earlier in this book, left me with back issues for the rest of my life. However, stretches, exercise, and strengthening the Erector Spinae muscle along my spine has helped to keep the pain in check.

Your body keeps its balance by combining information from these three key systems:

- **Vestibular System:** Located in your inner ear, this system senses head movements and changes in motion or direction. Tiny hair cells in the ear detect shifts in the fluid, letting your brain know which way you're tilting or moving.
- **Visual System:** Your eyes observe the environment around you. By noticing things like the horizon or nearby objects, they help your brain understand where you are and how you're moving.
- **Proprioceptive System:** This system comes from sensors in your muscles, joints, and skin that continuously report the position and movement of your limbs. It lets your brain know exactly how your body is positioned in space.

The brain takes all these signals, processes them, and then sends commands to your muscles to adjust your posture. This coordination helps you stand, walk, and move without falling over.

Your posture is key. Good posture gives you good balance. If you are hunched over, your weight is forward. It sets you up for falling forward.

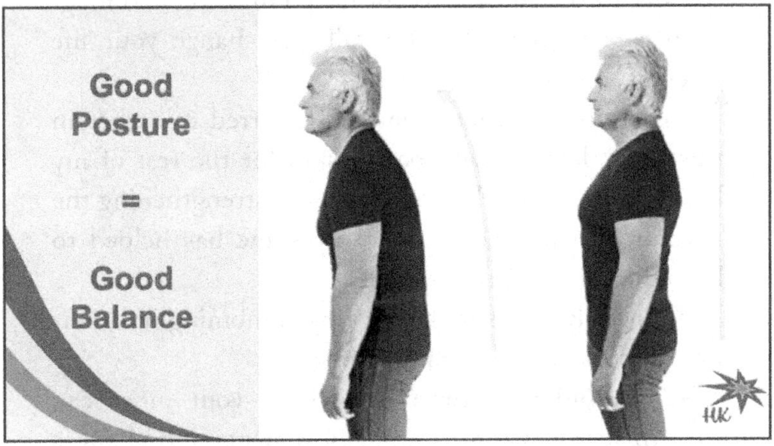

Good posture is when your shoulders are over your hips, and your hips are over your heels.

Here is what you can do to get into the perfect posture:

- Stand up, lift your shoulders up, push them back, and release them down. This should line your shoulders up with your hips. This may feel like you are sticking your chest out. That is because you have been slouching over and good posture doesn't feel natural (yet!).
- Then tighten your core muscles. Yes, you have muscles under the belly fat. Tighten them to improve your balance.

I work on posture with all my clients to help with their balance. I tell them shoulders back, tighten your core so much that they hear my voice in their head.

I had a client who said he was slipping on the ice. His hands were flying everywhere and his feet were sliding. He said it was worthy of a youTube video. Then he heard my voice in his head say, "shoulders back, tighten your core" and that is what he did and was able to regain his balance immediately. He told the class that story one day. It works!

Strong core muscles will help you maintain good balance. Yes, exercise and strength training come in to play again. It is important to strengthen your core to help with your balance.

There are some simple activities you can do at home to improve your balance. Remember if you don't use it, you'll lose it.

Do these balance activities daily. Set a time of day when you do them. In the morning while you are waiting for your coffee to perk or when you are waiting for the microwave to finish isn't a bad time since you have a minute or two.

Standing on one leg.

Stand next to something steady that you can hold on to (kitchen counter, chair without wheels, wall). Get into the perfect posture (shoulders back, tighten your core) then lift one knee up bringing your foot off the ground. Try to balance on one leg for 15 seconds. Then do the same for the other leg.

Tandem Standing

Stand next to something steady that you can hold on to (kitchen counter, chair without wheels, wall). Get into the perfect posture (shoulders back, tighten your core), place the heel of the front foot in front of the toes of your back foot. Hold that position for 15 seconds, then switch feet and hold for 15 seconds.

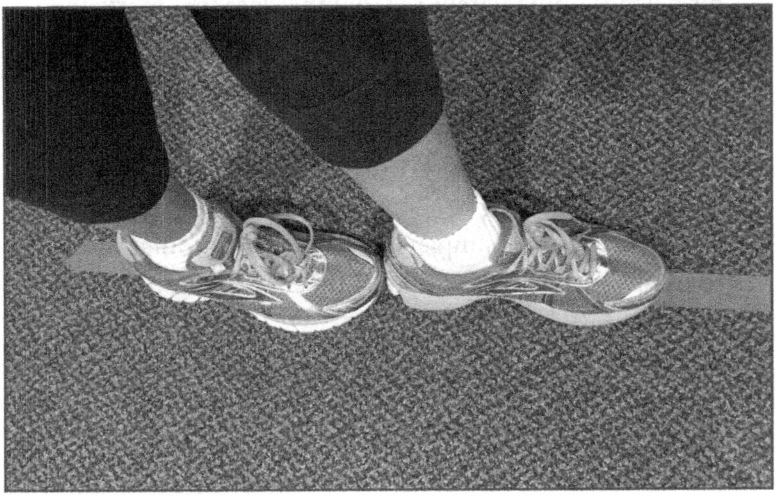

Tandem Walking

For tandem walking, it may be easier if you put a piece of painter's tape on the floor so you can walk the line. If you don't have tape, you can walk the tile line if you have tiles in your kitchen, or walk the plank if you have wood floors (just don't go overboard).

Stand next to something steady that you can hold on to (kitchen counter, chair without wheels, wall). Get into perfect posture (shoulders back, tighten your core), place the heel of the front foot in front of the toes of your back foot. Walk forward always keeping the heel of your front foot touching the toes of your back foot. Once you have mastered this, then walk backwards using tandem walking. Keep reminding yourself, shoulders back, tighten your core to keep your balance.

Once you have improved your balance, you can try more challenging balance activities using balance devices like a balance disc.

You can also practice standing on one leg with your eyes closed (hold on to something steady like a chair). Since your visual system is part of helping you to balance, when you take that away, you challenge your body more to balance. **Only practice standing on one leg with your eyes closed if you are already proficient in balancing on one leg.**

Other activities you can do to improve your balance are yoga or Tai Chi. These activities work on balance. Taking a yoga or Tai Chi class can make a big difference in your balance and can be very relaxing as well.

Brain

I have already shown you the studies that show when you improve your balance you will improve your cognitive abilities and when you improve your cognitive abilities, you will improve your balance.

Let's talk about how your brain needs resistance training and overload just like your muscles do. Regular mental and physical exercises will increase your brain's response time and your cognitive abilities.

Resistance training for your brain is doing new and challenging cognitive activities.

For example, if you always do crossword puzzles, your brain is not engaging in a new activity. You need to change it up and do something different like Sudoku or a jigsaw puzzle. If you always read a certain genre of book, then change it up and read something totally different. Maybe try reading a fantasy book to get your brain actively working to comprehend what you are reading.

Play games like bridge, mahjong, monopoly, trivial pursuit, or scrabble. As I mentioned earlier in this book, I play mahjong every week with a group of ladies. It is a nice brain challenge, as well as a fun social event.

Solving puzzles and brainteasers will activate your brain in ways that are different than your everyday thinking.

There are several Apps you can play on your phone or online to challenge your brain. I use Elevate and Lumosity. They are fun and challenging.

Search Apps on your phone for brain games and give them a try.

Exercise and Your Brain

As you can see from the picture below that certain types of physical activities activate different parts of the brain. You can improve function in different parts of the brain with exercise.

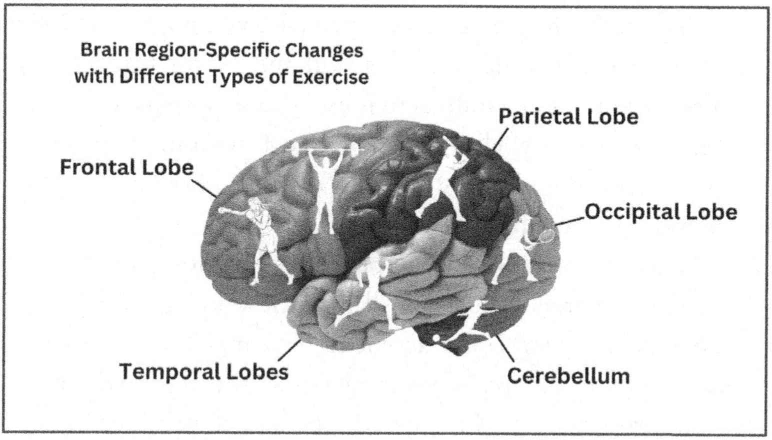

The **Frontal Lobe** can be affected by doing cognitive demanding activities like resistance training and Mind - Body exercises. What these activities do for the frontal lobe is increase the gray matter in the brain, improve executive functions, and give you more efficient brain activity.

The **Parietal Lobe** can be affected by doing sensory rich activities and activities with visual spatial demands. These activities will improve the white matter and volume of the parietal lobe, improve sensory network activity, and improve the ability to switch between tasks more easily.

The **Occipital Lobe** can be affected by doing activities with visual spatial demands, visual attention demands, and motor control and stimulation activities. These activities will increase the white and grey matter of the occipital lobe, improve visual skills and attention, and increase volume and function of the occipital lobe.

The **Cerebellum** can be affected by doing coordinative exercises, that requires skill and motor learning, along with open skill activities. These activities will increase the cerebellum volume and function, improve coordination and attention, and increase nerve cell and blood vessel volume.

The **Temporal Lobe** can be affected by doing cardiovascular exercise, closed skill activities, and generalize physical activity. These activities will improve learning and memory, increase Neurogenesis (the regrowth of new brain cells), and increase hippocampal volume.

These were just summaries. Now I will get into more specifics on the types of exercises and their effect on the different parts of the brain.

Frontal lobe

The frontal lobe is one of the most crucial areas of the brain, playing a key role in our "executive functions." These are the primary roles of the frontal lobe:

- **Executive Functions & Decision-Making**
  It's involved in planning, problem-solving, and decision-making, helping us set goals and determine the steps needed to achieve them. This includes regulating our behavior, controlling impulses, and adapting to new situations.
- **Motor Control**
  The frontal lobe houses the primary motor cortex, which is essential for initiating and controlling voluntary movements. It also includes regions that

plan and coordinate more complex motor actions like dancing or golf.

- **Language Production**
  In most people, the left frontal lobe contains Broca's area, a region critical for speech production and language processing.
- **Social Behavior & Personality**
  The frontal lobe helps shape our personality and social interactions. It guides our ability to understand social norms, empathize with others, and manage emotional responses.
- **Working Memory & Attention**
  This area also supports working memory—the ability to hold and manipulate information over short periods—and helps maintain focus and attention during tasks.

In summary, the frontal lobe is vital for a range of higher-order processes that enable us to plan, move, communicate, and interact socially, making it central to our daily functioning and overall behavior.

Here are several types of exercise that have been linked to improvements in the frontal lobe:

Aerobic Exercise

(Running, brisk walking, cycling, swimming)

- Aerobic activities increase blood flow to the brain, promoting the release of growth factors such as brain-derived neurotrophic factor (BDNF). This helps with the growth and maintenance of neural connections in the frontal lobe, enhancing executive functions.

- Studies indicate that regular aerobic exercise can lead to improvements in attention, processing speed, and overall cognitive flexibility.

Resistance Training

(Weight lifting, bodyweight exercises, resistance band workouts)

- Strength training not only improves physical health but also influences brain health. It may reduce inflammation and improve insulin sensitivity, both of which are beneficial for maintaining neural health and cognitive function.
- Some research has shown that resistance training can help improve planning and problem-solving abilities, particularly in older adults.

Mind-Body Exercises

(Yoga, Tai Chi, Qigong)

- These exercises combine physical movement with mindful awareness and controlled breathing. They help reduce stress and anxiety, which can impair cognitive functions. The improved stress management from these activities support better regulation of the frontal lobes executive processes.
- The coordination and balance involved in these activities also contribute to better neural connectivity and overall brain health.

Coordination and Dual-Task Training

(Dancing, martial arts, sports that require split-second decision-making)

- Activities that require simultaneous physical movement and cognitive engagement (such as remembering choreography or responding to opponents in sports) challenge the brain to coordinate complex motor actions with decision-making. This dual-task nature can stimulate the frontal lobe, enhancing cognitive flexibility and working memory.
- These exercises engage both the motor and cognitive domains, encouraging the brain to develop more robust neural networks.

Incorporating a mix of these exercise types into your routine can provide a comprehensive boost to executive functions in your frontal lobe. Aerobic exercise improves overall brain blood flow and growth factor release; resistance training supports neural health through metabolic benefits; mind-body practices reduce stress while promoting balance and coordination; and complex activities that require dual-tasking can challenge and thereby enhance the cognitive processes tied to executive functioning.

By regularly engaging in these varied forms of exercise, you're not only taking care of your body but also actively supporting your brain's ability to plan, focus, and adapt.

Parietal Lobe

The parietal lobe is a key hub in the brain for processing and integrating sensory information. Here's what happens in this region.

- **Spatial Awareness and Navigation:**
  The parietal lobe plays a crucial role in helping you understand where objects are in space relative to your body. This ability is essential for tasks like navigating through an environment or reaching for objects.
- **Integration of Sensory Information:**
  Beyond just receiving sensory data, the parietal lobe integrates information from multiple senses to create a comprehensive picture of your surroundings. This integration supports coordinated movement and perceptual accuracy.
- **Attention and Perception**
  It contributes to the allocation of attention, ensuring that you can focus on specific aspects of your environment while filtering out irrelevant stimuli.

  By analyzing spatial relationships and sensory details, it helps in recognizing and categorizing objects.
- **Higher Cognitive Functions**
  Some parts of the parietal lobe are involved in processes like reading, writing, and performing mathematical calculations, linking sensory inputs to more abstract cognitive tasks.

In summary, the parietal lobe acts as a central processing station for sensory data and spatial information, ensuring that you not only feel your environment but also understand and interact with it effectively.

Enhancing parietal lobe functioning through exercise generally involves activities that challenge spatial awareness, sensory integration, and coordination. While most forms of physical activity benefit overall brain health, these exercises may particularly stimulate the parietal lobe:

Aerobic Exercises with Spatial Demands

(Running or cycling in different environments or hiking on uneven terrain)

- Aerobic exercise increases overall blood flow and supports neuroplasticity, while navigating new or variable environments forces you to continuously process spatial information and adjust your movements accordingly.

Balance and Coordination Training

(Yoga, Pilates, Tai Chi, Balance Board exercises)

- These activities require maintaining equilibrium and precise body control, which improves sensory integration and proprioception—the sense of where your body is in space. These types of exercises directly challenge the parietal lobe by requiring continuous adjustment based on sensory feedback.

Dual-Task and Complex Motor Activities

(Choreographed movement, Martial arts, Basketball or Soccer)

- Exercises that combine physical movement with cognitive demands (for instance, tracking a moving ball or following a dance sequence) force the brain to integrate multiple streams of sensory information. This multi-tasking helps sharpen spatial awareness and coordination, which are key functions of the parietal lobe.

Obstacle Courses and Interactive Training

(Interactive video games, virtual reality programs designed to challenge spatial navigation, obstacle courses)

- These activities require you to interpret sensory data quickly and plan your movements accordingly, reinforcing neural networks in the parietal cortex that are responsible for processing complex spatial relationships.

While no single exercise targets the parietal lobe exclusively, incorporating activities that involve aerobic movement in varied environments, balance and coordination challenges, and dual-task exercises can collectively support the sensory integration and spatial processing functions of this brain region. Regular engagement in these exercises not only improves physical fitness but also promotes neuroplasticity and cognitive health.

I have mentioned **neuroplasticity** several times and I want to give you the definition of neuroplasticity also called neural plasticity. According the Merriam-Webster dictionary, **neuroplasticity** is the brain's ability to form and reorganize synaptic connections, especially in response to learning, experience, or following injury. Basically, it is a process that shapes and molds different parts of the brain to take on new functions.

Occipital Lobe

The **occipital lobe** is the part of the brain primarily responsible for visual processing. It is located at the back of the brain and plays a crucial role in interpreting and making sense of the information received from the eyes.

These are the main functions of the Occipital Lobe:

- **Visual Processing & Recognition**
  It interprets signals from the retina to form images and helps recognize faces, objects, and colors.
- **Depth Perception & Spatial Awareness**
  It determines how far objects are and their relationship to each other, which is important for activities like driving, sports, and hand-eye coordination.
- **Color & Motion Perception**
  It distinguishes colors and movement patterns. The occipital lobe is essential for tracking moving objects and recognizing changes in the environment.

- **Reading & Visual Interpretation**
  It helps recognize letters, words, and symbols. It also supports reading comprehension and pattern recognition.
- **Visual Memory & Imagination**
  Assists in recalling visual images and forming mental pictures. It plays a role in creativity and visualization exercises.
- **Integration with Other Brain Areas**
  The occipital lobe works with the parietal lobe for spatial awareness. It communicates with the temporal lobe for object and facial recognition. It interacts with the frontal lobe to guide decision-making based on visual input.

The occipital lobe is primarily responsible for visual processing, so exercises that engage and challenge visual perception, coordination, and memory can help keep it active. Here are some activities that specifically stimulate the occipital lobe:

Visual Processing Exercises

- Spot the Difference: Find differences between two similar images.
- Puzzles & Optical Illusions: Engaging with complex images or ambiguous figures strengthens visual processing.
- Where's Waldo & Hidden Object Games: These improve visual scanning and attention.

Eye-Hand Coordination Activities

(Ping Pong, Tennis, Racquet Ball, Squash, Pickleball)

- Juggling: Improves visual tracking and coordination.
- Ball Toss Games: Catching and throwing exercises strengthen spatial awareness.
- Ping Pong or Tennis: Fast-paced sports requiring visual tracking.

Color & Shape Recognition

- Sudoku & Pattern Games: Enhance recognition of colors, patterns, and spatial relationships.
- Drawing or Painting: Engages visual creativity and hand-eye coordination.

Peripheral Vision Training

(soccer, basketball, agility ladder)

- Soccer & Basketball: Enhances visual-motor coordination, peripheral vision, and reaction time.
- Agility Ladder: Step through a speed ladder in various patterns (sideways, hopping, high knees) while focusing on foot placement.

Spatial Awareness and Smooth Eye Movements

(Tai Chi, Qigong)

- Tai Chi: Improves balance, spatial awareness, and smooth eye movements.

- Tai Chi & Qigong: Perform slow, controlled movements while keeping your gaze focused on your hand movements or a distant point.

These activities help the Occipital lobe improve visual-spatial processing and the brain's ability to anticipate movement. They also boost coordination between vision and movement, reducing strain on the occipital lobe.

Cerebellum

The cerebellum is responsible for balance, coordination, motor control, and precise movement. Physical exercises that challenge these functions can enhance cerebellar activity, which will improve motor skills, reaction time, and cognitive function.

Here are some exercises that stimulate the cerebellum:

Balance Training

(Enhances Stability & Coordination)

- Tandem Standing & Walking as described earlier in this book.
- Standing on one leg, progress to closing your eyes (always have a chair or stable surface available to hold on to).
- Standing on an unstable surface (e.g., Balance Disk or BOSU ball) – this is more advanced (always have a chair or stable surface available to hold on to).

Coordination Drills

(Strengthens Motor Control & Timing)

- Cross Crawls: Lift your right knee and touch it with your left elbow, then switch. Repeat for 1-2 minutes. This exercise can be done on the floor lying face down or standing.
- Finger-to-Nose Test: Close your eyes, extend your arm, and touch your nose with your finger.

Agility Ladder Drills

(Boosts Reaction Time & Spatial Awareness)

- Step through a ladder pattern quickly (side steps, high knees, or crossover steps). Keep your head up and focus on moving efficiently.

Dance & Rhythmic Movement

(Improves Motor Learning & Memory)

- Dance to music with varied tempos. Try complex footwork patterns or partner dancing for added challenge.

Martial Arts or Tai Chi

(Develops Precision & Motor Adaptability)

- Practice slow, controlled Tai Chi movements or basic martial arts drills. Focus on transitioning smoothly between positions.

By consistently practicing these exercises, you can strengthen cerebellar function, leading to better balance, smoother movement, and improved motor learning.

Temporal Lobe

The temporal lobe is responsible for memory, language, auditory processing, and recognizing faces & emotions. Engaging in physical exercises that incorporate sound, rhythm, coordination, and memory can strengthen its function.

Here are some exercises that stimulate the temporal lobe:

Dancing

(Memory, Rhythm & Coordination)

- Try Zumba, ballroom, or hip-hop dance.
- Learn a new dance routine and recall it without watching a video.

Yoga with Deep Breathing & Chanting

(Mind-Body Connection & Auditory Processing)

- Try Humming Breath (inhale deeply, then exhale while humming).
- Hold poses like Tree Pose or Warrior Pose while mentally recalling a short phrase or song.

Walking While Listening to Audiobooks or Conversations

(Language Processing & Comprehension)

- NOTE: Only use one ear bud or ear piece so that you are still aware of your surroundings while walking.
- Listen to a podcast, audiobook, or song lyrics while walking. Try repeating key points or lyrics afterward.

Tai Chi or Martial Arts

(Reaction Speed & Cognitive Function)

- Follow a Tai Chi routine, focusing on slow, controlled movements.
- Practice shadowboxing with an emphasis on remembering movement patterns.

Memory-Engaging Cardio

(Cognitive Challenge While Exercising)

- While jogging or cycling, recite numbers or a story in your head.
- Try a "countdown game" where you name backwards sequences (e.g., 100-3-97-3-94…).

In summary to boost your temporal lobe, engage in rhythmic activities (dancing, drumming, Tai Chi), combine movement with auditory tasks (listening to podcasts while walking), and incorporate memory challenges into exercises (naming objects while playing catch).

Improvements in your temporal lobe will also improve learning & memory, increase Neurogenesis (the regrowing of new brain cells), and increase hippocampal volumes. The hippocampus is where your memory is stored.

White Matter versus Grey Matter in the brain

I have referenced the white and grey matter of the brain several times. Let me explain in easy terms what they are and what they do.

Your brain has **two main types of tissue: grey matter** and **white matter.** Think of them like the hardware and wiring of a computer—both are essential for the brain to function properly.

Using the computer analogy:

Grey Matter = The Brain's Processing Center

- It processes information, makes decisions, and controls movement, memory, and emotions.
- It is found on the outer layer of the brain (cerebral cortex) and deep inside in important areas like the hippocampus (memory center).
- Think of it as the computer's processor (CPU) — it does the thinking, learning, and problem-solving.

White Matter = The Brain's Wiring System

- It connects different parts of the brain, allowing grey matter regions to send messages to each other quickly.
- It is found deep inside the brain and spinal cord, forming "communication highways."
- Think of it as the internet cables or electrical wires—it helps different brain areas work together smoothly.

If the computer analogy doesn't work for you, try thinking of it like a city.

Using a city analogy:

Grey matter = The buildings

- Where thinking and decision-making happen (schools, offices, houses).

White matter = The roads and highways

- They connect the buildings so messages can travel efficiently.

Without grey matter, you wouldn't be able to think, move, or feel emotions.

Without white matter, your brain wouldn't be able to send messages fast enough to function properly.

As we see in several of the areas of the brain, certain activities can increase the grey and/or the white matter in that area of the brain.

What other things can you do to keep your brain sharp?

The brain needs resistance training and overload just like your muscles.

Regular mental and physical exercises will increase your performance and cognition.

However, you need to do new and challenging things.

As we mentioned when discussing activities to improve function in your Occipital lobe, brain games will help keep you sharp.

These activities help to train your brain:

- Play games like scrabble, monopoly, battleship, mahjong, and card games.
- Do crossword puzzles, word search, sudoku, and jigsaw puzzles.
- Read books of different genres to let your brain experience new scenarios.
- Play some brain games on your computer or phone to speed your reaction time, better your comprehension, and improve your problem-solving skills. Some brain game websites: Luminosty.com, Fitbrains.com, BrainHQ.com.

Social Interaction

Socialization plays a crucial role in maintaining and enhancing brain function. Engaging in regular social interactions has been linked to better cognitive health, reduced risk of dementia, and overall improved mental well-being. Here are some key findings from recent studies:

- **Cognitive Benefits of Social Engagement:** Research indicates that individuals who are more socially connected tend to live longer and enjoy better physical, mental, and cognitive health outcomes. Social activities stimulate various cognitive functions, potentially delaying or preventing cognitive decline. [10]
- **Impact on Dementia Risk:** A 2023 meta-analysis of 13 longitudinal aging studies, encompassing nearly 40,000 participants, found that individuals with regular social connections had a lower risk of developing dementia. This suggests that social engagement may serve as a protective factor against cognitive decline. [11]
- **Brain Aging and Social Interaction:** Studies have shown that social interaction doesn't just enhance mood but also helps to slow down brain aging. Engaging in social activities has been associated with reduced cognitive decline as we age. [12]

In summary, maintaining an active social life is essential for brain health. Regular social engagement supports cognitive functions, reduces the risk of dementia, and contributes to overall mental well-being.

I encourage you to stay socially active. Don't stay home by yourself. I know my dad found it hard to go and do social activities with others after my mom passed away. For some reason he felt that people who went to the Senior Center were old. In reality, because he stayed more isolated, he was the old one.

Stay active with others to keep your mind sharp and maintain good mental health.

You can look for resources that have activities you can participate in. Your town may have a Council on Aging or a Senior Center where you can attend classes, luncheons, go on day trips, or to the movies, etc. Stay active with others to keep your mind sharp and maintain good mental health.

Music and your Brain

My sister-in-law asked me to do some research on music and brain health.

I found multiple studies that suggest that playing a musical instrument in later life is associated with better memory, stronger executive function, and slower cognitive decline.

Playing a musical instrument certainly is a positive lifestyle habit. It fits nicely alongside other brain-healthy behaviors (physical exercise, social engagement, learning new skills). It also may involve socialization while playing the instrument that adds to the benefits.

While it's not guaranteed to prevent dementia, playing an instrument is a low-risk, rewarding activity that appears to build cognitive reserve. It is never too late to learn to play an instrument.

Key Points

- Good posture is good balance! Push your shoulders back and tighten your core to help your balance. Practice balance activities daily. If you don't use it, you lose it!
- Use your brain in different ways to keep sharp. If you consistently do crossword puzzles, change it up and do a jig saw puzzle or Sudoku. Your cognitive abilities increase when you challenge your brain.
- When you improve your balance, you improve your cognitive abilities. When you improve your cognitive abilities, you improve your balance.
- Exercise is important for your brain to function well. Cardio exercise will help your memory. Strength training will help executive function. You can improve function in the different lobes of the brain with different type of exercise.
-

Staying socially active keeps your brain sharp.

Personal Thrive Formula
Brain & Balance

When you increase your balance, you increase your cognitive abilities.

What activities do you do NOW to activate your brain?

____

____

What activities can you add to your life to keep your brain young?

1. ______________________________________

2. ______________________________________

3. ______________________________________

4. ______________________________________

What activities do you do NOW to improve your balance?

____

____

What activities can you add to your life to improve your balance?

1. ______________________________________

2. ______________________________________

3. ______________________________________

4. ______________________________________

Stay Socially Active!

Putting it All into Action

Don't be the person who can't get up off the toilet alone!

Exercise so climbing stairs or standing up from a chair doesn't feel hard to do!

Choose to be stronger! Make the changes necessary to remain independent and functional longer in your life.

You have learned how important it is to add exercise to your day. Be sure to build some muscle not just for strength but also to increase your metabolism. Go for a walk, it is one the best exercises you can do.

Start to eat healthier foods. Put the junk food down. If you want a healthy body, you need to feed it healthy foods.

Start to incorporate some of what you learned from this book into your lifestyle today. You now understand how important it is to stay active, eat healthy foods, keep your brain engaged, and to continuously work on your balance.

Set a goal to add one new habit each week. Work on the habit for a whole week before you add another habit.

These are the four simple habits I recommend you incorporate into your lifestyle:

- Drink more water (48-64 oz/day)
- Take a walk (15-30minutes) every day
- Do 20 Push-ups a day
- Practice Tandem Walking daily

Once these habits are incorporated into your lifestyle you can move on to lifestyle changes like eating healthier foods. Make sure you take at least a week for each new habit to make it stick. While you are adding a new habit, don't let the others slip off. Build on (or stack habits) a habit each week. If you start to feel overwhelmed, take a few weeks for each new habit.

These simple steps will help you feel energized and healthy.

If you find yourself stuck and not able to add these healthy habits, contact me through my website and I will give you some Holly's Helpful Hints to help you get started.

I know you can do it! You just need to start.

TODAY!

Glossary

Active Ager — A person (in the later stages of life) who prioritizes physical, mental, emotional, and social well-being to lead a fulfilling and engaged lifestyle.

All-Cause Mortality — The overall death rate from any cause, regardless of the specific reason for death.

Alzheimer's Disease — Alzheimer's disease is a progressive, neurodegenerative disorder that primarily affects the brain, leading to memory loss, cognitive decline, and behavioral changes.

Atrophy (Muscle Atrophy) — The wasting away or decrease in size of muscle tissue.

BMR (Basel Metabolic Rate) — The energy your body uses when your body is at rest.

Blue Zones — Areas where people live longer than other areas of the world.

Cardio Vascular Exercise — (Also known as aerobic exercise or "cardio,") refers to physical activities that increase the heart rate, breathing rate, and blood flow throughout the body.

Cerebellum — The Cerebellum, located at the base of the brain at your neck, is responsible for balance, coordination, motor control, and precise movement.

Dual Task Training — Activities that require simultaneous physical movement and cognitive engagement at the same time.

Dynamic stretching — Moving through a range of motion with controlled movements.

EAT (Exercise Activity Thermogenesis) — The energy used during an exercise workout (a gym class or a structured workout).

Exercise — Organized session of moderate-to-intense physical activity usually lasting about 30 minutes or longer.

Erector Spinae — A group of muscles that run along the spine, responsible for extending and laterally flexing the vertebral column. They are also crucial for maintaining posture and stability.

Fibrous Carbohydrates — Complex carbohydrates that are rich in fiber, a type of indigestible carbohydrate that plays a crucial role in digestion and overall health.

Flexibility — Increasing the range of motion at joints by stretching muscles. Essentially it is making your body more flexible.

Frontal Lobe — The frontal lobe, located in the front of the brain, is one of the most crucial areas of the brain, playing a key role in our "executive functions."

Genetics — The study of how genes and traits are passed down from one generation to the next.

Grey Matter — Processes information, makes decisions, and controls movement, memory, and emotions. It is found on the outer layer of the brain (cerebral cortex) and deep inside in important areas like the hippocampus (memory center).

Healthspan — Healthspan is how many years you remain healthy and free from disease.

Insulin Resistance (or Sensitivity) — The cells in your muscles, fat, and liver don't respond well to insulin. If your cells don't respond well to insulin, over time your pancreas may not make enough insulin to help extra glucose enter your cells.

Hippocampus — The part of the brain where your memory is stored.

Lifespan — Lifespan is the total number of years we live.

Lifestyle — The typical way of life of an individual.

Life Expectancy — The average lifespan of an individual.

Longevity — Length of life.

Metabolism — The body's way of using food to fuel its activities, growth, and maintain its health.

MIND Diet — (Mediterranean-DASH Intervention for Neurodegenerative Delay) is a combination of the Mediterranean and DASH (Dietary Approaches to Stop Hypertension) diets that focuses on protecting brain health and reducing the risk of cognitive decline.

Movement — Any intentional or unintentional effort to move your body.

Muscle Mass — The total amount of skeletal muscle tissue in the body.

NEAT (Non-Exercise Activity Thermogenesis) — The energy used when you are doing non-exercise activity throughout the day.

Neural Connectivity — The intricate network of connections between neurons in the brain, enabling communication and information processing.

Neuroplasticity — The capacity of the brain to develop and change throughout life, something Western science once thought impossible.

Nutrition — The act or process of nourishing or being nourished. It is the foods you eat to nourish your body.

Occipital Lobe — The Occipital Lobe, located below the Parietal Lobe at the lower back of your brain, is primarily responsible for visual processing. It plays a crucial role in interpreting and making sense of the information received from the eyes.

Osteoblasts — Osteoblasts are cells that are responsible for creating new bone.

Osteoclasts — Osteoclasts are cells that dissolve bone tissue, also called bone resorption.

Osteoporosis — Osteoporosis is a disease that causes bone density and mass to decrease, leading to weaker and more fragile bones.

Parietal Lobe — The Parietal Lobe, located behind the Frontal Lobe, is a key hub in the brain for processing and integrating sensory information.

Pilates — A type of exercise and body conditioning that emphasizes core strength, controlled breathing, and muscle engagement, enhancing muscle tone and stability. It is done on specific equipment and/or on the floor.

Piriformis Muscle - The piriformis is a small, pear-shaped muscle located deep in your buttock, behind the gluteus maximus. It runs diagonally from the lower spine to the outer hip.

Posture — The position in which someone holds their body when standing or sitting.

Proprioceptive Neuromuscular Facilitation (PNF) — A stretching technique that utilizes muscle contractions to enhance stretching effectiveness. Holding a muscle tight for a period of time and then releasing it to increase its flexibility.

Proprioceptive System — This system comes from sensors in your muscles, joints, and skin that continuously report the position and movement of your limbs. It lets your brain know exactly how your body is positioned in space.

Protein — Any food that provides a significant amount of protein, an essential nutrient your body needs for building and repairing tissues, for making enzymes and hormones, and supporting overall health.

Qigong — An ancient Chinese practice that focuses on cultivating and directing qi, which is often translated as "life force" or "vital energy." It combines mindful movement, breathing exercises, and meditation to promote physical, mental, and spiritual well-being.

Sacroiliac Joint Dysfunction — Abnormal motion in the sacroiliac joint, either too much motion or too little motion, that causes pain in this region.

Sarcopenia — The loss of muscle mass, strength, and function (generally in older adults).

Sciatica — Nerve pain that travels along the path of the sciatic nerve, which runs from the lower back down the leg.

Starchy Carbohydrates — A type of carbohydrate that contain a high amount of starch, a complex carbohydrate that provides the body with energy.

Static Stretching — Holding a stretch for a sustained period of time.

Strength Training — (Also known as resistance training) is a type of exercise that involves using weights or body weight to improve muscle strength and endurance.

Tai Chi — A mind-body exercise combining slow, flowing movements, focused breathing, and meditation. It originated as a martial art in China but has evolved into a practice focused on promoting health and well-being.

Tandem standing — Also known as a tandem stance, is a balance exercise where you stand with one foot directly in front of the other, heel to toe.

Tandem Walking — Also known as heel-to-toe walking, is a balance exercise where you walk in a straight line with the heel of one foot placed directly in front of the toes of the other foot.

TEF (Thermic Effect of Food) — The energy used in the digestion and storage of the food we eat.

Temporal Lobe — The Temporal Lobe, located in front of the Cerebellum and touches all the other lobes of the brain, is responsible for memory, language, auditory processing, and recognizing faces & emotions.

Total Daily Energy Expenditure (TDEE) — How your body burns the calories you consume.

Vegan Diet — A diet that is exclusively plant based and does not contain any foods that come from animals (no dairy, meat, eggs, or honey).

Vestibular System — Located in your inner ear, this system senses head movements and changes in motion or direction. Tiny hair cells in the ear detect shifts in the fluid, letting your brain know which way you're tilting or moving.

Visual System — The biological system that enables us to see and interpret our surroundings. It encompasses the eyes, the optic nerve, and the visual cortex in the brain, all working together to process visual information.

White Matter — Connects different parts of the brain, allowing grey matter regions to send messages to each other quickly. It is found deep inside the brain and spinal cord, forming "communication highways."

Yoga — Uses body postures that focus on flexibility, body awareness, and a mind-body connection. It includes breath control and simple meditation that is widely practiced for health and relaxation.

End Notes

Chapter 1

1. Li Y;Pan A;Wang DD;Liu X;Dhana K;Franco OH;Kaptoge S;Di Angelantonio E;Stampfer M;Willett WC;Hu FB; "Impact of Healthy Lifestyle Factors on Life Expectancies in the US Population." Circulation. Accessed October 19, 2025.

   https://pubmed.ncbi.nlm.nih.gov/29712712/.

2. Morris MC;Tangney CC;Wang Y;Sacks FM;Bennett DA;Aggarwal NT; "Mind Diet Associated with Reduced Incidence of Alzheimer's Disease." Alzheimer's & dementia : the journal of the Alzheimer's Association. Accessed October 19, 2025.

   https://pubmed.ncbi.nlm.nih.gov/25681666/.

Chapter 2

3. Diagram Credit: http://www.joedavis.com.au
4. Volpi, Elena, Reza Nazemi, and Satoshi Fujita. "Muscle Tissue Changes with Aging." Current opinion in clinical nutrition and metabolic care, July 2004.

   https://www.ncbi.nlm.nih.gov/pmc/articles/PMC2804956/.

   Holloszy JO. The biology of aging. Mayo Clin Proc. 2000 Jan;75 Suppl:S3-8; discussion S8-9. PMID: 10959208.

   Melton LJ 3rd, Khosla S, Crowson CS, O'Connor MK, O'Fallon WM, Riggs BL. Epidemiology of sarcopenia. J Am Geriatr Soc. 2000 Jun;48(6):625-30. PMID: 10855597.

Chapter 3

5. "Phil Kaplan - Body Transformation Program." Phil Kaplan. Accessed October 19, 2025.

   https://philkaplan.com/.
6. Pearson, Keith. "The Mind Diet." Healthline, February 7, 2025.

   https://www.healthline.com/nutrition/mind-diet#meal-plan.

Chapter 4

7. Volume 72 issue 4 | The Journals of Gerontology: Series A | Oxford academic. Accessed October 19, 2025.

   https://academic.oup.com/biomedgerontology/issue/72/4.

8. Rogge, Ann-Kathrin, Brigitte Röder, Astrid Zech, Volker Nagel, Karsten Hollander, Klaus-Michael Braumann, and Kirsten Hötting. "Balance Training Improves Memory and Spatial Cognition in Healthy Adults." Scientific Reports 7, no. 1 (July 18, 2017).

   https://doi.org/10.1038/s41598-017-06071-9.

9. Li Y;Pan A;Wang DD;Liu X;Dhana K;Franco OH;Kaptoge S;Di Angelantonio E;Stampfer M;Willett WC;Hu FB; "Impact of Healthy Lifestyle Factors on Life Expectancies in the US Population." Circulation. Accessed October 19, 2025.

   https://pubmed.ncbi.nlm.nih.gov/29712712/.

10. "Social Connection and Brain Health." Social Connection and Brain Health - Memory and Brain Wellness Center. Accessed October 19, 2025.

    https://depts.washington.edu/mbwc/news/article/social-connection-and-brain-health.

11. SEO, StudioHawk. "The Link between Social Connections and Brain Health." SFI Health, March 21, 2025.

https://www.sfihealth.com/news/the-link-between-social-connections-and-brain-health.

12. "How Social Connection Keeps Your Brain Young: Study." UNSW Sites. Accessed October 19, 2025.
https://www.unsw.edu.au/newsroom/news/2022/10/how-social-connection-keeps-your-brain-young--study.

Photo Credits

All photographs © Holly Kouvo, unless otherwise noted.

Image licensed from Shutterstock (Image ID:2211549359, *retirement-couple-running*) used under standard editorial license.

Image licensed from Shutterstock (Image ID: 590135870, *basket-of-veggies*) used under standard editorial license.

Image licensed from Shutterstock (Image ID: 580617103, *middle-age-man-reading-book*) used under standard editorial license.

Image licensed from Shutterstock (Image ID: 390767452, *Senior man on his mountain bike*) used under standard editorial license.

Image licensed from Shutterstock (Image ID: 236053966, *Senior Man Using Walking Frame,*) used under standard editorial license.

Image licensed from Shutterstock (Image ID: 520248718, *Senior couple exercising in gym,*) used under standard editorial license.

Image licensed from Shutterstock (Image ID: 2280496733, *Painful Struggle An Overweight Woman Suffers with Leg Pain at Home*) used under standard editorial license.

Image licensed from Shutterstock (Image ID:486631567, *Spanish Steps in Square of Spain*) used under standard editorial license.

Image licensed from Shutterstock (Image ID: 2472675723, *Senior couple, kayak and rowing,*) used under standard editorial license.

Image licensed from Shutterstock (Image ID: 1056228761, *Grandparents Running Along Beach,*) used under standard editorial license.

Image licensed from Shutterstock (Image ID: 228796489, *elderly man in winter snowshoeing,*) used under standard editorial license.

Brit Huckaby, *Julia Hawkins BHM2017,* licensed for use by author, 2025

Image licensed from Shutterstock (Image ID: 1894312669, *Ill senior woman making inhalation at home,*) used under standard editorial license.

Image licensed from Shutterstock (Image ID: 2441747477, *group-exercising-arms-out-front-stretching,*) used under standard editorial license.

Image licensed from Shutterstock (Image ID: 2117309684, *piriformis_syndrome,*) used under standard editorial license.

Image licensed from Shutterstock (Image ID: 2476905077, *healthy-food,*) used under standard editorial license.

Image licensed from Shutterstock (Image ID: 2159311389, *stack-of-wood,*) used under standard editorial license.

Image licensed from Shutterstock (Image ID: 1904696305, *Burning firewood in fire-box,*) used under standard editorial license.

Image licensed from Shutterstock (Image ID: 718803511, *middle-age-man-crossing-log-bridge,*) used under standard editorial license.

Image licensed from Shutterstock (Image ID: 1439827739, *senior-man-posture,*) used under standard editorial license.

Image licensed from Shutterstock (Image ID: 2280979459, *brain-colored-lobes,*) used under standard editorial license.

Image licensed from Shutterstock (Image ID: 653015995, *male runner,*) used under standard editorial license.

Image licensed from Shutterstock (Image ID: 1694309644, *Male lifter,*) used under standard editorial license.

Image licensed from Shutterstock (Image ID: 2110748537, *soccer player female,*) used under standard editorial license.

Image licensed from Shutterstock (Image ID: 2153139957, *baseball player,*) used under standard editorial license.

Image licensed from Shutterstock (Image ID: 2237913655, *female boxer,*) used under standard editorial license.

Image licensed from Shutterstock (Image ID: 2410171683, *tennis player woman,*) used under standard editorial license.

Resources

American Association of Retired Professionals
www.aarp.org

American Heart Association
www.Heart.org

American Society on Aging
www.asaging.org

Fitting Fitness In
www.FittingFitnessIn.com

Institute on Aging
www.ioaging.org

National Council on Aging
www.ncoa.org

National Institute on Aging
www.nia.nih.gov

ABOUT THE AUTHOR
Holly Kouvo

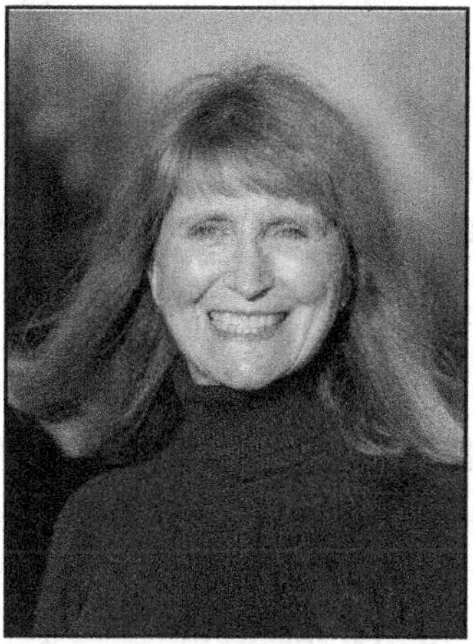

Holly Kouvo is passionate about reigniting the lives of aging Americans through simple fitness shifts that help them retain their independence and increase their daily joy. She is an instructor, coach, writer, media resource, and public speaker who lives the lessons she teaches, and always finds a way for Fitting Fitness In®, which is also the name of her company.

A fitness instructor for 30+ years and the proprietor of her own personal training company for over 20, Holly is waging war on unnecessary aging brought on by sedentary lives, poor nutrition, and a lack of hope or vision about the possibility of an active life at age 80 and beyond.

Holly has a BA from State University of New York at Potsdam. She is a certified Brain Health Trainer and Functional Aging Specialist by the Functional Aging Institute, Nutrition Specialist by the American Academy of Sports Dietitians and Nutritionists, Personal Trainer and Aerobics Instructor by the Aerobics and Fitness Association of America.

Holly has published articles in several national magazines, including *American Fitness* and *IDEA Fitness Journal,* and has been a regular contributor to several health, fitness and active lifestyle websites including Martha Stewart's Wholeliving.com. Holly released her first exercise DVD called "Total Body Workout...Just Easy on The Knees™" in the fall of 2006. In addition, she had a weekly radio spot, "Holly's Helpful Hints", on Career/Life Balance Radio (WNRI.com).

Over two million households nationwide follow "Get Healthy with Holly" on cable access television. Holly is an author of multiple books, a health coach to online clients, and teaches exercise classes online, and in person.

When she's off the clock, Holly Kouvo loves her life among the apple trees of Stow, MA and can be seen through the kitchen window doing squats as she makes her family dinner.

Holly speaks on many topics pertaining to health, wellness, fitness, nutrition, brain health, balance, and active aging.

Learn more about Holly at
www.HollyKouvo.com.